ON BEING VEGAN:

Reflections on a
Compassionate Life

by Colleen Patrick-Goudreau

No book can replace the diagnostic expertise and medical advice of a trusted physician. Please be certain to consult with your doctor before making any decisions that affect your health, particularly if you suffer from any medical condition or have any symptom that may require treatment. Published in the United States by Montali Press.

The Joyful Vegan® is a registered trademark of Colleen Patrick-Goudreau

Copyright © 2013 Colleen Patrick-Goudreau
All rights reserved.
ISBN: 0615787215
ISBN 13: 9780615787213

Cover design by Aaron Weinstein
Cover photo by Sara Remington

PRAISE FOR ON BEING VEGAN

"Colleen Patrick-Goudreau has once again managed to pack a small, easy-to-read volume with invaluable insights that are enlightening for both new and longtime vegans. Even though I've been active in the vegan movement for over 20 years and have written my own books on the subject, *On Being Vegan* provided me with new wisdom and a deeper level of personal empowerment. ~*Melanie Joy, Ph.D., Author of* Why We Love Dogs, Eat Pigs, and Wear Cows *and President and Founder of the Carnism Awareness and Action Network*

"With her unending wealth of knowledge, insightful personal experience, and authentic affection for her readers, Colleen Patrick-Goudreau offers this deeply engaging manifesto on just about everything the conscious consumer ponders in a way that everyone can digest." ~*Jasmin Singer, Executive Director of Our Hen House*

"With *On Being Vegan*, Colleen Patrick-Goudreau demonstrates once again why she is a leading voice in the worldwide movement toward a more compassionate way of living. Drawing on her years of experience as an animal activist, vegan cookbook author, podcast producer, cooking instructor, public speaker, and confidante, Colleen explores what it means to live a fully awakened life—a life steeped in an abundance of choices, flavors, and new experiences. Whether you're a longtime vegan or thinking of taking the leap, you'll find *On Being Vegan* to be a healthy helping of commonsense advice and myth-busting. ~*Mark Hawthorne, author of* Striking at the Roots: A Practical Guide to Animal Activism *and* Bleating Hearts: The Hidden World of Animal Suffering

"Colleen Patrick-Goudreau is a visionary. She translates vegan ideals into accessible prose and practice more effectively than any animal advocate I know. The fact that she does so through the seductive conceits of cooking, eating, and personal narration allows her authentic voice of compassion to echo across a divide too often marked by acrimony and confusion. Relentlessly positive, her message will intuitively appeal to vegans, almost-vegans, and no-way-I'd-ever-be vegans alike, which is to say: all of us." ~James McWilliams, vegan advocate, blogger, and author of *A Revolution in Eating* and *Just Food*

"As veganism continues its unremitting expansion into our culture, there are few working as persistently and creatively as Colleen Patrick-Goudreau to help people understand the profound benefits of vegan living, and what it actually is. In *On Being Vegan*, she provides a solid foundation for

both the theory and practice of vegan living, and covers, in a concise and readable way, the immense breadth of veganism as well as how it affects the details of daily life. In it, she brings her characteristic thoughtful and empowering perspective that has endeared her to so many people searching for guidance and clarity in their quest for living more compassionate, healthy, and aware lives. Highly recommended."
~Will Tuttle, Ph.D, author of the acclaimed best-seller, *The World Peace Diet*, is a pianist, composer, Dharma Master in the Zen tradition, and joyful vegan since 1980.

ALSO BY COLLEEN PATRICK-GOUDREAU

* Vegan's Daily Companion: 365 Days of Inspiration for Cooking, Eating, and Living Compassionately

* Color Me Vegan: Maximize Your Nutrient Intake and Optimize Your Health by Eating Antioxidant-Rich, Fiber-Packed, Color-Intense Meals That Taste Great

* The Vegan Table: 200 Unforgettable Recipes for Entertaining Every Guest at Every Occasion

* The Joy of Vegan Baking: The Compassionate Cooks Traditional Treats and Sinful Sweets

* The 30-Day Vegan Challenge: Online Life-Changing Multimedia Program

DEDICATION

To David, my amazing husband and fellow joyful vegan, whose unshakable support and unconditional love form the foundation on which I stand.

TABLE OF CONTENTS

AUTHOR'S NOTE TO READER

Thank you so much for picking up *On Being Vegan: Reflections on a Compassionate Life*. The essays contained within address the core aspects of what it means to be vegan.

* In the first chapter, I recount my own personal story from compassionate child to desensitized adult.

* Chapter 2 comprises the origins of the word "vegan," its definition, and its meaning, as I understand it.

* Chapter 3 provides an overview of some of the most compelling reasons people choose to leave animal products off their plates.

* In Chapter 4, I detail the tangible and intangible benefits of living free of animal products, taking great care to empower you with the information you need to measure your own success.

* Chapter 5 offers a guide for deciphering labels, helping you to recognize the most healthful, animal-free ingredients.

* Chapter 6 answers some questions that people tend to ask when they begin thinking about the ethical considerations of animal use and consumption.

* In Chapter 7, I emphasize that being vegan is about doing the best we can in our imperfect world – not about worrying that the vegan police will come knocking on your door.

The topic of veganism is massive, as it touches every aspect of our lives, and this book is just the first in a multi-volume endeavor. My hope is that the content herein provides a foundation on which you can begin to build your own story.

As you enjoy this volume and await (hopefully) the next one, I invite you to explore my other works and books, including:

* my online multimedia program, The 30-Day Vegan Challenge: provides everything you need to make the vegan transition confidently, healthfully, joyfully, and deliciously. 30DayVeganChallenge.com

* my podcast, Vegetarian (it's vegan!) Food for Thought: addresses every issue related to being

vegan, including food, cooking, nutrition, animal rights, family dynamics, food politics, and social psychology – and debunks the myths surrounding these issues. It's free and available on iTunes, on my website, and at VegetarianFoodForThought.com

* my cookbooks *The Joy of Vegan Baking, The Vegan Table, Color Me Vegan* and inspirational book, *Vegan's Daily Companion*. Available everywhere books are sold.

* my website: recipes, resources, videos, and everything you need to live compassionately and healthfully. CompassionateCook.com

Thank you for letting me be part of your journey. I'm so glad we're on this ride together.

— Colleen Patrick-Goudreau

CHAPTER 1:

A JOURNEY TO AWAKENING

I was raised in a typical American family eating the typical American fare: anything that walked, swam, or flew. My father owned ice cream stores, and we had a separate freezer to store the gallons he brought home. Veal Parmesan was a common menu item in our house and in local restaurants, Chicken a la King was my favorite dish, and I drank chocolate (cow's) milk with abandon. I didn't necessarily choose these foods. They were chosen for me. Nobody told me what they were made from, and when I asked, my parents and the adults around me either evaded the question entirely or deceived me completely.

I was also typical in that I cared very deeply about animals. I'm reluctant to say I "loved animals," because I don't believe you have to *love* animals to *not want to hurt them*, but I did (and do) *adore* animals. I loved being around them,

I had no fear of them, and I intervened and wept whenever I saw them suffering. When a bird fell in our yard with an injured wing, I built a little house for her until she was well enough to fly again. When homeless dogs made their way to our doorstep, I brought them in until I found their people. When my mother took me to see the movie *Benji*, I wept until I wailed when the little dog Tiffany was kicked by a cruel human.

I remember the day we adopted our dog, a little gray Schnauzer with floppy ears and a loud, persistent bark. The first few nights away from her littermates, she cried and whimpered until I convinced my mother to let me hold her while she fell asleep. I don't think I loved animals more than most children do, and my parents and the adults around me supported and encouraged this compassion in every way.

Images of baby animals adorned all of my clothing, wallpaper, and bedding; animal cut-outs hung over my crib in a musical mobile; and stuffed animals were my constant companions in and out of my bed. I sang songs about animals and played games where I mimicked animals; I was brought to the zoo to admire animals; and on many a Halloween, I dressed up as animals. More than that, animals were used to teach me my most fundamental skills through characters in books and television shows who taught me how to count, how to spell, how to read, and how to talk. Through the use of myths and fables, animals even taught me such values as respect and kindness, and I learned social mores through their teachings.

In every aspect of my life, I was given the message that non-human animals were integral to who I was – even shaping who I was becoming.

But what I didn't know – because nobody told me – is that I was being fed the dismembered bodies of animals – the very same animals I was brought to the zoo to pet. The very same animals whose wings I helped mend. The very same animals whose faces were depicted on my pajamas.

And so I was taught – implicitly, of course – to categorize animals into arbitrary and paradoxical compartments of those we love and those we eat, those we live with and those we exploit, those worthy of our compassion and those undeserving of it because they happen to be of a particular species or bred for a particular use. In other words: puppies good, calves food. The message I received was that the injured bird who was lucky enough to fall into my yard was worth saving, but the chickens and turkeys whose lives "sacrificed themselves so that I might eat them" were valuable only in so far as their flesh was tender and juicy. In other words: chickadees friends. chickens dinner.

At the same time, I was also learning to compartmentalize and temper my compassion. I was given the message that life is not always fair and nature is not always kind but that God put animals on the earth for us to eat and that I should be grateful for His kindness and their sacrifice. That fierce, unconditional compassion I had as a child began to become dulled, as my taste for animal flesh and fat began to grow and settle into my palate.

The good news is that though my innate unconditional compassion was put to sleep, it didn't disappear. As I grew up and continued to consume whatever came off of or out of an animal, I'm aware that there was a great sense of discomfort always lurking within my conscience. I made excuses, I justified my choices, and I pretended that labels depicting "happy animals" absolved me of any pangs of guilt I might have felt.

Luckily, when I was 19 or 20 years old, I picked up *Diet for a New America* by John Robbins, and the course of my life changed forever. This was the first book to examine the effects of our animal-based diet on our health, on the environment, and on the animals themselves, and it was certainly the first time I had ever seen the images of animal factories, where lives are regarded as machines and the value of the animals determined only by what they produce. I stared at photos of hens in cages with the tips of their beaks seared off, female "breeding" pigs confined in crates the size of their own overgrown bodies, turkeys packed in windowless sheds, calves chained to boxes. I remember staring at those images in utter shock. How could I not have known about this? How could I have contributed to it? How could this even happen? I knew didn't want to be part of it, so I stopped eating land animals that very day.

Interestingly, my parents and other adults around me didn't quite react the same way they had as when I was a child. Helping fallen baby birds or taking in stray animals were considered admirable childhood pursuits and met with support and admiration, but when that very same compassion – no different in substance or strength – followed me into adulthood and extended to pigs, cattle, chickens, and other animals killed for human consumption, it was greeted with hostility and suspicion. The message was: Limited compassion: good. Unconditional compassion: bad. Childhood compassion: normal. Adult compassion: extreme and sentimental.

Nonetheless, my awakening had begun, and I was not deterred. I was, however, still partially asleep. I had stopped eating land animals, was learning everything I could about these issues, and had begun raising awareness and advocating for animals, but I continued to consume chicken's eggs, cow's milk, and aquatic animals. This lasted for several years until I was knocked into full consciousness while reading *Slaughterhouse: The Shocking Story of Greed, Neglect, and Inhumane Treatment Inside the U.S. Meat Industry* by investigative journalist Gail Eisnitz. I will never forget how incredibly painful it was to read this book and how incredibly powerful it was to feel my eyes and heart opening. Becoming fully awake was a visceral, cleansing, heart-rending process, and I wouldn't change it for all the world, however many tears I shed in the few days it took me to read the book.

The lens through which I saw the world changed, and the paradigm by which I lived my life completely shifted.

I came to fully comprehend that no matter how animals are raised or what they are raised for (their flesh, eggs, or milk), in the end, it's all the same, and that end is a nightmare. After reading John Robbins' book, I would have said that I stopped eating land animals (I didn't identify as a "vegetarian" because I was still consuming fish) because I didn't like the way they were treated. But after reading *Slaughterhouse*, it became much more rudimentary than that. I became aware of how wasteful, unnecessary, and absurd it is to bring animals into this world only to kill them. I became utterly offended at how we manipulate the reproductive system of females for their milk, capitalizing on their ability to give birth only to take her young from her and impregnate her again. I became fully aware of the violence inherent in breeding, keeping, transporting, and killing animals for our pleasure and uncomfortable that I was complicit in paying people such as those who work in slaughterhouses to become desensitized to their own compassion and to the animals' suffering.

It was as if I had been sleepwalking up until then. Granted, I had been participating in life and experiencing fulfilling relationships, but simply put, I was not *really* living my life according to my own values. If you had asked me if I perceived myself as a compassionate person, I would have said "absolutely!" But, in truth, my actions were not in sync with my self-perception. I would never have intentionally hurt another living being, and yet I was paying others to do it for me. Reading the personal accounts of slaughterhouse workers who abused, dismembered, tortured, and killed animals literally shook me out of my slumber. Once awake, I couldn't but act, and the natural response was to stop participating in this system.

I "became vegan" overnight.

I'm struck by how funny that phrase can sound. We say a caterpillar "becomes" a butterfly or a seed "becomes" a flower and can easily imagine what they look like in their transformation. But what does it look like to "become vegan"? Prior to becoming awake, I had been practicing selective compassion. "Becoming vegan" was my metamorphosis into embracing my unconditional, unfettered, unabashed compassion. That is to say, my deepest ethics became reflected in my daily choices, and the process was as natural and effortless as is the process for a caterpillar to become a butterfly or a seed to become a flower.

I'm tempted to say that I returned to the unconditional compassion of my childhood, but I don't think that's the entire truth of it. When I was a child, I acted compassionately *without* any thought – as if I didn't know any better than to respond to those who needed my help. It just came naturally. As an awakened adult, I act compassionately *with* thought, and I regret only that the innocent kindness of a child is valued more than the informed kindness of an adult.

Despite the fact that compassion is a guiding principle in all the world's religions and even in secular philosophies, the primary message we receive by the time we're adults is that compassion is acceptable as long as it is *conditional*, reserved only for certain groups/species. And though we admire compassion in children, we're taught to be somewhat *suspicious* of compassionate adults. Operating within these boundaries of selective compassion, how can we not feel a weight on our minds and in our hearts?

This process of turning innately compassionate children who identify deeply with animals into desensitized adults who participate in the exploitation of animals is universal and, I argue, profoundly detrimental. I believe that it is this process that fundamentally keeps us from being fully whole, fully complete, fully enlightened human beings.

After all, how can we be fully complete human beings having hardened a part of our hearts? How *can* we be fully complete having put to sleep a central aspect of who we are? How can we be fully complete if we avoid looking at certain things lest they be too painful to face or live in fear that the truth might reveal our own complicity? How can we be completely whole if we create boundaries to our compassion?

When we turn away from the reality of what we do to animals for our gustatory pleasure, we play a game of pretend, like the child who covers her eyes and thinks you can't see her. And yet, there she remains. Closing our eyes doesn't make violence disappear; it only closes our minds and hearts and enables the violence to continue. It was only when I was willing to *look* at how I contributed to violence against animals that I became awake, and in doing so, I have not so much returned to the innocent compassion of my childhood but instead have found a deeper place – where my eyes and heart are open not because of what I *don't* know but because of what I *do* know.

CHAPTER 2:

DEFINING VEGAN

Although the word "vegan" has gained traction in the public consciousness, on restaurant menus, on food packaging, and in the media in recent years, misunderstandings and misconceptions still prevail about what "vegan" means. Some who call themselves "vegan" eat animals such as chickens and fish; some eat what are marketed as "free-range eggs"; and others who call themselves "vegan" eat animal products when it's convenient for them or when they eat out or travel.

So, first, let's define what "vegan means.

In the most literal sense,

* to be "vegetarian" means to eat anything but the *flesh* of animals, whether those animals walk, swim, or fly.

* to be "vegan" means to eat or wear anything but the flesh *and* secretions of animals, which includes anything that comes out of or off of an animal, such as their hair, fur, skin, milk, and eggs.

But veganism goes well beyond this literal definition; it is a tangible manifestation of abstract principles, and it is a powerful way to live. The word itself was coined in 1944 by British activist Donald Watson, who lived from 1910 to 2005. He was born in Yorkshire in the northern part of England, and as you might imagine, intentional vegetarianism – let alone veganism – was not exactly popular in the farming and meat-eating community in which he grew up.

In interviews, Watson recounts his early childhood memories of seeing animals pushed through doors alongside butchers' shops to be killed. He talks about the time he saw a cow and a calf enter together and wondered later which one the butcher killed first. On another occasion, he watched a cow being killed at an abattoir (slaughterhouse) in a field where local children could see and hear it all happening. And he talks about spending time at his Uncle George's farm, where various animals were kept. He remembers that

> they all "gave" something: the farm horse pulled the plough, the lighter horse pulled the trap, the cows "gave" milk, the hens "gave" eggs and the cockerel was a useful "alarm clock." The sheep "gave" wool. I could never understand what the pigs "gave,"

but they seemed such friendly creatures – always glad to see me. Then the day came when one of the pigs was killed: I still have vivid recollections of the whole process - including the screams, of course. One thing that shocked me was that my Uncle George, of whom I thought very highly, was part of the crew. I decided that farms - and uncles - had to be reassessed: the idyllic scene was nothing more than Death Row, where every creature's days were numbered by the point at which it was no longer of service to human beings.[1]

And so Watson made the very conscious decision to stop eating animals as a New Year's resolution, and it stuck for 81 years. 18 years after he became vegetarian, he became vegan. He was 32 years old, and it was 1942. His brother and sister eventually joined him, and though their parents were initially concerned about potential health risks, their fears proved to be unfounded.

Dedicated to this compassionate way of living, Watson went on to help form The Vegan Society (vegansociety.com), the first vegan organization in the United Kingdom, in 1944. By this time, an organization called "The Vegetarian Society" was already in existence, having been founded in Kent - in South East England - in 1847. This group was the first to popularize the word "vegetarian," and they claim to have created the word from the Latin *vegetus*, meaning "lively," though the Oxford English Dictionary states that "vegetarian" was formed from the word "vegetable." Whatever the origins of the word, the fact is that Donald Watson had become disheartened by the fact that "vegetarianism," a diet that originally excluded *all* animal products, came to embrace some of these very things.

And so, Donald asked members of his burgeoning organization to come up with a more concise word to characterize vegetarians who ate no animal products. The suggestions he received ranged from the literal – "dairyban" – to the creative – "vitan," "benevore," and "sanivore" – but ultimately he and his wife, Dorothy, decided on the word "vegan" by taking the first three and last two letters of "vegetarian," because, as Watson explained, "veganism starts with vegetarianism and carries it through to its logical conclusion."

The word and its definition were accepted by the Oxford English Dictionary, and though the word has certainly caught on, especially in recent years, it seems the pronunciation still has not. Watson himself, however, was clear about how it is pronounced, insisting that it is VEE-gun – not VAY-gun, VEE-jun, or VAY-jun.

Donald didn't merely coin the word (and clarify its pronunciation); he also created a very precise and beautiful definition. Watson defined veganism as "a philosophy and way of living which seeks to exclude—as far as is possible and practical—all forms of exploitation of and cruelty to animals for food, clothing, or any other purpose."

Based on Watson's definition, "being vegan" is about making conscious, compassionate choices; it is not about trying to attain an impossible level of purity or striving to become a 100% certified vegan. There is no such thing—our world is simply too imperfect for that. Even Watson acknowledges this in his definition when he qualifies: "*as far as is possible and practical.*"

I think one of the reasons people tend to equate veganism with perfection is because they're operating under the misconception that being vegan is an *end* in itself. But being vegan is not an end; it's a *means* to an end. And for me, that end is optimal wellness and unconditional compassion: reflecting our highest selves by doing everything we can to make choices that cause the least amount of harm – both to ourselves and to others. Being vegan is a powerful and effective means toward attaining that end, but it is not the end itself.

"Vegan Food" is Normal Food

In the many years I've been doing this work, what I know for sure is that people want to make healthful and compassionate choices, but they also want these choices to be convenient and familiar, and they assume being vegan is neither.

It's no surprise we have these misconceptions about veganism. We are taught early on in our culture that meat, dairy, and eggs are "normal" foods for regular folks and that "vegan food" is unsubstantial and lacking, reserved for "health freaks" or for the allergy-prone. Unfortunately, these misperceptions lead people to believe that many of their familiar favorites are not vegan.

And so let's set the record straight here and now:

Bread is vegan. It's true that some brands and types of commercial breads have animal's milk added to them – but certainly not all. Good bread – real bread – is naturally vegan. Just think of the definition of bread according to French law: "it can contain nothing more than flour, salt, water and yeast."

Pasta is vegan. Although some types of pasta have chicken's eggs added to them – namely *egg* noodles – by definition, pasta is really just made from flour and water. In fact, the word originally meant "pastry dough sprinkled with salt."

Chocolate is vegan. One of the biggest misconceptions about being vegan is that you have to forego chocolate, having to settle only for carob. Au contraire! By definition, chocolate is a plant-based food; it comes from the cacao tree. Cocoa butter, cocoa powder, bittersweet chocolate, semi-sweet chocolate, dark chocolate, even white chocolate, are all vegan by nature. Only when you add cow's milk (or any animal's milk) is chocolate not vegan. Some companies play with definitions by adding cow's milk to what they label semi-sweet and dark chocolate bars and chips, but by definition, semi-sweet and dark chocolate do not contain cow's milk. That's what I mean when I say they're playing with definitions. When shopping for chocolate, just take a quick peek at the ingredients to make sure there is no added "milk fat," "milk powder," or "casein," and choose higher quality brands.

Cocoa *butter* is vegan. We tend to associate the word *butter* with dairy, but really it has more to do with *fat* than animal's milk. Peanut *butter*, cocoa *butter*, coconut *butter*, almond *butter*, shea *butter* – are all plant-based fats. Cocoa butter is simply the fat in the cacao bean, so just because a label says "butter" doesn't mean it contains an animal product.

Vegans eat yeast. Considering the fact that yeasts are microorganisms classified as fungi (not animals), of course vegans eat yeast, which means, as I said: bread is vegan.

When you get down to it, "vegan food" is food we already cook with and already love. We just might not call it "vegan." If you've had an apple, you've had "vegan food." If you've ever eaten spaghetti with marinara sauce, you've had "vegan food." We don't say "vegan apple" or "vegan banana." We know these foods are vegan because they're real, whole foods!

When we stop distinguishing "vegan food" from "regular food," we recognize that "vegan food" is food that we're all familiar with – it's vegetables and fruits, nuts and seeds, grains and legumes, mushrooms and sea vegetables, herbs and spices. In the case of baked goods, it's flour, sugar, cocoa, chocolate, vanilla, spices, baking soda, baking powder, cornstarch, and yeast.

When we take these foods out of the box called "vegan," we recognize that they're not so unfamiliar after all, and we begin to see how expansive our choices are.

Changing our Perception

I've heard every excuse in the book for not going vegan, and I'm certain that each one stems from fear-based perceptions rather than experiential reality. This is evident in some of these common excuses:

* *Cooking vegan food is very different and much harder than cooking meat and animal products.*

* *I tried being vegan, but I got bored with eating the same food over and over again. I wanted more options.*

* *If I become vegan, I'll experience restriction, limitation, and deprivation.*

The problem is that our perception of ourselves and our habits isn't always aligned with reality. As William Shakespeare said – through Hamlet – [There is] "nothing either good or bad, but thinking makes it so."

If you've been looking in one direction your whole life, choosing the same foods over and over, and not stretching any comfort zones, you're most likely stuck in habits and routines that compel you to make snap judgments against "vegan food," placing it in an ugly box marked "other" and allowing yourself to remain unchanged.

And yet, if you think about the process of going from eating Italian cuisine your whole life to learning how to prepare Indian cuisine, you're intuitively aware that you'll need to learn some new techniques and explore some new ingredients, but you don't *judge* Indian cuisine for being *inferior* to Italian cuisine. You just recognize that it's different and unfamiliar to *you*.

The same holds true when we transition to becoming vegan. Although many foods will certainly be familiar (vegetables, fruits, grains, nuts, etc.), you become aware of how many more food choices there are than ever before. It's not that those choices weren't available to us when we were eating meat, dairy, and eggs; it's just that we weren't looking outside of our comfort zone. When we shift our gaze from one direction to another, an entirely new world opens up – one full of new cuisines, new flavors, new textures, new aromas, and new experiences. And how exciting is that? Isn't it wonderful that there is so much to learn and so many new things to explore?

Re-Envisioning Our Plates

Some of our blocks about veganism aren't really about the food itself but about *how* we plate our food. In our meat-centric culture, we're accustomed to having a piece of animal-based meat at the center of our plate surrounded by some token vegetables, most likely covered in dairy-based butter and fat-laden cream sauces. Many people perceive a "vegan meal" as lacking because they imagine that piece of meat being removed – leaving the plate half-empty with only "side dishes" remaining.

But the way we plate our food is merely a cultural habit – what we've been taught in our families and in our society. If you think about various cuisines around the world and how the food is plated, you'll remember that it looks very different from our typical Western meal. Think of Indian, Mexican, Thai, Chinese, Vietnamese, Japanese,

Middle Eastern, or Ethiopian cuisines. The plates are made up of what we tend to call "side dishes," and yet these are the most healthful and flavorful foods, based on vegetables, grains, lentils, beans, and greens.

So, on the one hand, we need to rethink what a plate of food "should" actually look like as well as embrace the notion of filling our plates with what we have traditionally perceived of as "only side dishes."

However, I'm convinced that our attachment to having animal-based meat as the main dish has more to do with having a *focal point* on the plate than anything else, and there are many creative and beautiful ways to create a familiar-looking plate with a main dish and sides. With that in mind, we might try something stuffed (squash, eggplant, tomatoes, artichokes, or bell peppers) or something contained (such as mini pot pies or a timbale formed in a ramekin), or we might use something similar in texture and appearance to the animal-based meat we're accustomed to, such as mushrooms, tofu, tempeh, and seitan.

I'm not one to make promises to people about what they can expect when they "go vegan," but one thing I always guarantee is that over time, your palate definitely changes and expands. Most of us who grew up on meat, dairy, and eggs have insensitive palates virtually coated with fat and salt, nary able to detect the varied and subtle flavors of plant foods. But as you get these things out of your system, your palate becomes cleansed, and you become sensitized to things you never thought had flavor.

When you remain open, you experience changes you can hardly even anticipate.

Experiencing the Expansive

I'm not just encouraging you to be open to new foods. I'm encouraging you to be open to new perceptions and emotions. I've met my fair share of people who say "Eating vegan seems so limiting, so restrictive," and then in the same breath, they say something like "But don't tell me about how the animals are treated," they say. "I don't want to know. I don't want to see. I don't want to look." They might even literally cover their ears or their eyes.

How remarkable that we willingly *limit* knowledge and *restrict* awareness. In creating boundaries to our compassion and choosing ignorance over awareness, we deny ourselves the full experience of what it means to be human – feeling sorrow, as well as joy.

Now, I want to make it clear that I don't believe that people who avoid looking at animal abuse are insensitive to animal suffering; I believe they're *so* sensitive to it that it makes them close their eyes and subsequently their hearts. The very idea that animals suffer is so anathema to them, so difficult to confront – particularly if they're still eating them – that it's easier not to go there at all.

And yet, on a very personal level, every time we say, "Don't tell me. I don't want to know," we limit the potential for growth, for transformation, for making possible everything we want to be and everything we want this world to be. So we walk around with blinders on, complacent in our comfort zones because we're afraid to look, afraid to know, afraid to change. To me, *that's* limiting. *That's* restrictive.

On the contrary, being vegan is about being willing to know, willing to explore, willing to experience what is painful but true. Being vegan is about evolving, participating, and taking responsibility. To me, *that's* expansive. *That's* abundance.

Violence against animals is methodically and purposefully hidden from view because the animal exploitation industries know that the public is outraged and offended whenever they see the truth about what the animals endure. The worst thing we can do to the perpetrators and the best thing we can do for the animals is to uncover our eyes and bear witness to the abuses. Awareness is the greatest weapon against violence. Of course looking at the truth can be painful, but it's what many of us need to knock ourselves into consciousness and become part of the solution.

If you feel that watching something will hinder you rather than energize you, then be true to yourself. Learn where your line is, and be honest, but don't be so afraid of feeling sad that you avoid what is also a very human emotion. Being human, after all, is about embracing joy as well as sadness and anger.

All I ask is that we remain open. And when we do so, we experience countless and unexpected gifts of expanded awareness, expanded taste buds, and expanded hearts.

For me, being vegan is about living my life with integrity and compassion, knowing that every decision I make is done so with the intention of not contributing to the suffering and exploitation of non-human animals, or any-one for that matter. But it's about more than that, too. It's about creating joy, kindness, and meaning in a world so filled with violence and despair. Personally, I experience a palpable feeling of peace knowing that I am making a non-violent contribution to the world. Just as violence creates more violence, nonviolence also creates more nonviolence, and I like being on that side of the equation.

My perception that veganism is expansive compels me to gently correct people or forms that refer to it as a "dietary restriction" or a "special diet." When those opportunities arise, I cross out "restriction" and replace it with "abun-dance," and I assure them that being vegan is very "special" indeed.

Saying "Yes"

Another misconception about veganism is that there are *rules* about what vegans "can" and "cannot" eat. A scenario in which many vegans have found themselves involves someone who is enthusiastically talking about their favor-ite (non-vegan) recipe and then abruptly stops, turns to the vegan and says, "Oh, I'm sorry. You can't eat that." Or they start to offer a piece of candy and then say, "Oh – you can't eat that. I forgot. You're vegan." Or they start talking about a particular food and ask: "Can you eat that?" or "Are you allowed to eat that?"

Let's be clear: vegans *can* eat whatever we want. There's nothing we *can't* have. But there are some things we *don't want*. Making a choice to not put in our mouths the flesh and fluids that came off of or out of an animal's body is just that – a *choice*. It's not a matter of "can" and "cannot." We're "allowed" to have whatever we want. Nobody's stopping us. Meat, dairy, and eggs are not *illegal*. We don't follow a set of dietary laws.

It's not a matter of not being *able to*; it's a matter of not *wanting* to. We're not forbidden to eat animals. We don't *want* to eat animals.

I think the problem is that there is a perception that being vegan is about saying "no" – about declining things that are offered to us. It *appears* that being vegan is about deprivation and asceticism and sacrifice, and that's the problem – the *perception* of what it means to be vegan. If people are on the outside looking in, they tend to see what vegans *don't* choose. They don't see what we *are* choosing. And maybe some of that has to do with the fact that in public settings, in a world dominated by the animal-eating culture, people see vegans rejecting things far more than they see them embracing things.

But being vegan is not about rules or doctrine. It's not about restriction or self-denial. And though being vegan does involve saying "no" to some things – such as cruelty and exploitation and violence – at its core, being vegan is about saying "yes."

It's about saying "yes" to our values. What's the use in having values if they don't manifest themselves in our behavior? We say that someone who lives according to his or her values and ethics has integrity. Well, what does it mean to *not* manifest our values in our everyday behavior?

And how many of us actually translate our values into action? It's nice to say that we are kind, brave, caring, trustworthy, helpful people. It's nice to say that we're against violence and cruelty. Most of us are. But how many of us actually take these abstract values and put them into concrete action? For me, being vegan, which extends to every area of my life, is an opportunity to do just that: to put my abstract values into concrete action.

By choosing to eat life-giving rather than life-taking foods, I'm saying "yes" to my values of peace and nonviolence, of kindness, compassion, harmony, and simplicity.

By choosing to *look* at what is done to other animals – human and nonhuman – on my behalf, for my convenience, I'm saying "yes" to my values of accountability, of responsibility, of commitment to truth and knowledge.

By standing up for what I believe in and speaking on behalf of those who have no voice, I'm saying "yes" to my values of justice, courage, unity, and service to others.

My integrity as a human being is not separate from my values as "a vegan." In fact, the latter is an extension and reflection of the former.

This begs the question: can you fully manifest your values and *not* be vegan? I think it's a question each individual has to ask himself or herself, but speaking for myself, when I became vegan, all the guilt and hypocrisy I ever experienced disappeared, and any conflict I ever felt about who I *thought* I was and how I was actually living just melted away. In becoming vegan, my values and actions became synchronized. If you had asked me before I was vegan if I thought I was a compassionate person, I would have answered with a resounding "yes." I definitely considered myself compassionate, empathetic, and kind. But looking back, my perception of myself was not in alignment with my behavior. Paying people to do things to animals that I never would have been able to do myself is not a compassionate act. Supporting an industry that is in itself inherently violent is not a reflection of true compassion. It's not that there weren't areas in my life where I displayed compassion, but the fact is I wasn't immersed in the fullness of my compassion. How could I have been? I was supporting the very things that are antithetical to my core ethics. The very things Donald Watson witnessed on his uncle's farm were and are anathema to me:

* separating mothers from their babies

* bringing life into the world for the sole purpose of ending it

* valuing living beings not for who they are but for what use they can be to humans

* becoming so desensitized that you're able to kill and remain unmoved by the screams of your victims

Watson was no different than you or me in being repelled by violence. He reacted the way many before him reacted and the way many of us react today: his logical response was to stop participating in violence. And with all the talk today about how "small farms" are the answer to our discomfort with how animals are treated in animal factories, it's important to keep in mind that Watson was repulsed not by factory farming but by what takes place on small, local farms. He was 14 years young, and it was 1924. He didn't stop eating animals and their secretions because he witnessed a cold, mechanized system; he stopped eating animals and their secretions because he didn't want to be part of the inherently violent and unnecessary process of giving animals life only to use them up and cut them off (then cut them up). He saw animal agriculture for what it is: exploitative, ugly, messy, unpredictable, hard, cruel, and bloody – not as the romanticized thing we've made it out to be.

Something Big

Having coined the word "vegan," founded the first vegan organization, and dedicated his life to inspiring a compassionate world, Donald Watson was asked in an interview a few years before he died if he had any message for the millions of people who are now vegan.

His answer was this: "Take the broad view of what veganism stands for - something beyond finding a new alternative to scrambled eggs on toast or a new recipe for Christmas cake. Realize that you're on to something really big, something that hadn't been tried until 60 years ago, and something which is meeting every reasonable criticism that anyone can level against it. And this doesn't involve weeks or months of studying diet charts or reading books by so-called experts - it means grasping a few simple facts and applying them.

"We don't know the spiritual advancements that long-term veganism - over generations - would have for human life. It would be certainly a different civilization, and the first one in the whole of our history that would truly deserve the title of being a civilization."[2]

May you realize you are indeed onto something really big. It's up to each one of us to reflect our deepest values in our daily choices and, in doing so, create the healthful, compassionate world we all imagine. If not you, then who? If not now, then when?

CHAPTER 3:

WHY VEGAN? PICK A REASON – ANY REASON

U pon discovering someone is vegan, many people's first response tends to be, "Why are you vegan?" I think most vegans will say that though there may have been *one* thing that sparked their desire to be vegan, they remain so for a *number* of reasons. And there are as many reasons not to eat animals as there are lives that could be saved by making this simple dietary change.

Some people choose to stop eating animals and animal products to experience health benefits or to reverse a particular illness or ailment. Some people don't want to contribute to violence against animals or to pay people to work in an industry that necessarily desensitizes them to animal suffering and thus to their own compassion. Aware of the devastating effects of animal agriculture on the environment, some people are moved to help prevent global warming or global depletion in general. With precious rainforests disappearing in order to create grazing land for cattle, wild animals being killed at the behest of private ranchers, and precious resources (water, food, energy) being poured into what is an unsustainable system, eliminating the consumption of animal products is indeed a logical and sensible response.

Although I enjoy many health benefits from being vegan (high energy, low cholesterol, normal blood pressure, etc.), I became and remain vegan because I don't want to contribute to violence against animals. Upon becoming vegan, I immediately and unexpectedly felt a tremendous amount of peace knowing that the suffering of animals bred and killed for human consumption no longer has anything to do with me. Although I didn't expect anything radical to come of my decision to stop eating animals and their secretions, it has given me the deepest sense of serenity and clarity I could have ever imagined. My choices have increased, my perception has broadened, and my values have been strengthened. I have found no experience to be as profound as living my life in such a way that celebrates life, that finds divinity in every living thing, and that seeks to live as nonviolently, consciously, simply, and healthfully as possible.

So, pick a reason – any reason, and it alone would be good enough to justify eating an animal-free diet. And yet we have so many reasons. Whether you care about human rights, food safety, wild animals, the environment, world hunger, farmed animals, or your own health, just a cursory look at each social justice issue demonstrates how intricately linked they are to our consumption of animal-based meat, dairy, and eggs.

FOOD SAFETY

From age-old scourges such as smallpox and tuberculosis to threats like AIDS and SARS, our interactions with, farming of, and consumption of animals have always played a pivotal role as a source of human disease. Because we humans are physiologically similar to all other animals, we are susceptible to the wide range of bacteria, parasites, and viruses that infect the animals we eat. Though plant foods are subjected to exposure to bacteria, parasites, and other infectious agents, the biochemical makeup of plants is so different from ours that the microorganisms that infect them don't affect us. That's why you'll never meet a person with Dutch elm disease or aphids. If a plant food does contain an organism that threatens human health, then it's most certainly a contaminant from an animal source, usually through feces-contaminated irrigation water or feces from an animal who defecated directly on a crop. Unfortunately, whenever there's an outbreak of a foodborne illness that gets traced back to a plant crop, the media stop short of telling the whole story: that an infected animal is what contaminated the plant crop in the first place.

More than 250 diseases are transmitted through food[3], and these infectious microorganisms include salmonella, trichinella, toxoplasmosis, parasites, bovine spongiform encephalopathy (aka "mad cow"), hepatitis viruses, and cancer viruses. In the United States in 2011, an estimated 47.8 million people contracted a foodborne illness. Many cases go undiagnosed, and some are fatal[4].

WILD ANIMALS – ON LAND AND IN THE SEA

People who say they care nothing for farmed animals tend to declare themselves lovers of wildlife. What they may not know is that animals in the wild – both on land and in the sea – suffer immensely and die prematurely and often gruesomely because of our insatiable appetites for the bodies and secretions of domesticated animals. For nearly a century, the U.S. federal government has been involved in wildlife-killing campaigns designed to protect ranchers. The U.S. Department of Agriculture-led program Animal Damage Control (now euphemistically called Wildlife Services) spends millions of tax dollars each year to kill millions of coyotes, wolves, bears, mountain lions, birds, and many other animals as a subsidy for the agricultural and livestock industries. The U.S. government killed more than 3,752,356 wild animals in 2011[5], many at the request of farmers and ranchers.

When we turn to aquatic animals, we tend to have an interesting reaction. We may be okay paying people to kill fish on our behalf, but we have an emotional reaction when we hear about the death of "non-target" species – whales, dolphins, turtles, porpoises, and birds – also known as bycatch. Bycatch refers to animals unintentionally caught – and thus unwanted – by the fishing industry.

Commercial fishers use a number of techniques for ensnaring animals, from setting miles of line and baited hooks (called longlines) to catch animals such as sharks, swordfish, and tuna; to using large nets to catch schools of fish. These large nets are towed underwater by what are called trawlers. A trawler is a fishing vessel designed for the purpose of operating a trawl, a type of fishing net that is dragged along the bottom of the sea. In just one pass, a trawl can remove up to 20% of the seafloor flora and fauna[6], and the fisheries with the highest levels of bycatch are shrimp fisheries: 80%-90% of a catch may consist of marine species other than the shrimp being targeted. In addition, dredging along the ocean floor also breaks up coral and the habitats of bottom-dwellers. And because the same areas are dredged again and again, these habitats and inhabitants don't have time to recover before being destroyed again.

Every year, an estimated 100 million sharks and rays are caught and discarded. Many sharks die as a result of tuna fisheries, which have also had a high level of dolphin bycatch[7]. In addition to the millions of sharks we kill each year as bycatch, we also kill and up to 73 million sharks for their fins alone – for soup[8].

According to estimates from Duke University, which conducted a global study of the declining sea turtle populations that was published in 2004, more than 250,000 loggerhead and 60,000 leatherback turtles are snared each year by commercial longline fishing. Tens of thousands of these turtles die. The study's authors estimate that 3.8 million hooks were set each day in 2000, a total of 1.4 billion hooks from 40 countries for the year[9].

Another by-product of the fishing industry is the brutal death of baby seals. Because of the overfishing of cod by the Canadian fishing industry in eastern Canada – in the Atlantic Ocean for Newfoundland's northeast coast, the cod population declined to such a degree that the government stepped in in the late 1980s and imposed severe restrictions on commercial fishing. But it was too late. Because of overfishing, the fishery collapsed, never recovered (and never will), and the ecosystem changed such that it was no longer able to support codfish.

What does all this have to do with the seals, you ask? Scapegoating the seals for the collapse of the cod fisheries, fishermen demanded a kill. In 2003, the Canadian government bowed to pressure from the fishing industry and ordered the massacre of hundreds of thousands of seals, declaring war on the seals in hopes that massive seal kills will bring back the cod and keep their disgruntled fishermen working. In fact, cod is not a major food source of the harp and hood seal diet. Nonetheless, during the 3-year period of 2003-2005, the Canadian Department of Fisheries and Oceans (DFO) allowed a kill quota of 975,000 baby and adult harp seals and 30,000 adult hood seals[10]. When the "struck and lost" seals are included (these are the animals who've been hit but lost in the icy waters), the total killed exceeds one million, making this the largest marine mammal slaughter in the world[11].

THE ENVIRONMENT

However you look at it, raising animals for food is one of the leading causes of pollution and resource depletion today. The mega-tons of liquid and solid animal waste should be enough to inspire self-described "environmentalists" to turn away from animal-based foods. Contaminating the air, rivers, streams, and groundwater, animal urine and manure kill fish, create noxious fumes, and are major pollutants. According to a report published by the United Nations Food and Agriculture Organization (FAO), 37 percent of the pesticides used in the U.S. are to grow crops for animals raised for human consumption[12].

The livestock sector creates more greenhouse gas emissions as measured in CO_2 equivalent (18 percent) than transport. Read what Henning Steinfeld, Chief of FAO's Livestock Information and Policy Branch and senior author of the report, wrote: "Livestock are one of the most significant contributors to today's most serious environmental problems. Urgent action is required to remedy the situation."[13]

Eating "locally sourced meat," as some people recommend as a solution, does nothing to rectify the problem. The majority of the average household's carbon footprint doesn't come from *transportation* – that accounts for only 11%. It comes from *preparation*, and the preparation of meat is much more resource-intensive than that of plant foods[14].

If those reasons aren't enough:

* it's several times more efficient for humans to eat grains directly than to funnel them through farmed

animals, both in terms of the water used and the total outcome produced.

* petroleum oil fuels the thousands of miles of transportation to the feedlot, slaughterhouse, meat-packing plant, and supermarket.

* overfishing has depleted biodiversity in the oceans, and because aquafarms dump waste, pesticides, and other chemicals into ecologically fragile coastal waters, local ecosystems are destroyed, devastating animals and plants.

HEALTH

For some people, however, the direct effects of meat, dairy, and eggs on their health are what compel them to turn to a plants-only diet. As rates of heart disease, cancer, diabetes, hypertension, and other life-threatening conditions skyrocket in the United States, many researchers and medical experts come to the same conclusion: A vegetarian diet can help protect your health and even reverse some diseases, including the most common one—heart disease. Plant-based diets offer a number of nutritional benefits, including lower levels of saturated fat, cholesterol, and animal protein, as well as higher levels of carbohydrates, fiber, magnesium, potassium, folate, and antioxidants such as vitamins C and E and phytochemicals. Vegetarians have been reported to have lower body mass indexes than non-vegetarians, as well as lower rates of death from ischemic heart disease; vegetarians also show lower blood cholesterol levels; lower blood pressure; and lower rates of hypertension, type 2 diabetes, and prostate and colon cancer, according to the Academy of Nutrition and Dietetics (formerly the American Dietetic Association)[15].

WORLD HUNGER

We have no dearth of food on this planet. What we do have is a highly political system, an inequitable distribution system, and a worldwide increase in the consumption of meat, animal milk, and eggs. Almost 1 billion people in the world are starving, and a significant culprit is the animal agriculture system. By now, most people have heard that it can take up to 15 pounds of grain to produce just 1 pound of edible animal flesh – a pretty wasteful conversion[16]. What's more, because raising animals for human consumption creates a demand for crops that will be fed to farmed animals, animal agriculture is responsible for topsoil loss, soil erosion, and deforestation. More than half of the world's corn crop and more than 80% of its soybean crop are fed to farmed animals[17]. Because that is such an exorbitant amount of waste of food calories, even a 10% drop in U.S. meat consumption would make a significant difference in terms of food available to feed the world's starving millions.

VIOLENCE AGAINST FARMED ANIMALS

We have been taught to compartmentalize animals into those we eat, those who entertain us, those whose fur we take, those we keep in our homes, and so on. This social framework has divided up animals so that we can justify exploiting some but admiring or loving others. Most people would never think of killing the mourning doves they watch from their windows or the geese they feed at the park or the coyotes they glimpse in the wild. But because of our social and personal habits – not out of necessity – billions of animals are brought into this world solely to be killed. Some are used for years before they're sent to slaughter, but in the end, all are bred the same purpose – to be used for humans – and experience the same end – slaughter at a young age.

Not only is it not necessary, there is also nothing "natural" about animal agriculture. Breeding animals only to kill them is absurd at best, and killing animals when they're babies is standard – whether they're raised conventionally or in operations that are labeled "humane," "sustainable," "natural," "free-range," "local," "organic," "cage-free," "heritage-bred," "grass-fed," or "poetry-read." (Okay, the last one might not be an official term used, but it highlights the romanticism with which animal agriculture is marketed and regarded.)

*"Dairy cows" endure a constant cycle of pregnancy, loss, and forced lactation until their bodies are so worn out and depleted of calcium that they are sent to slaughter at 4 or 5 years young[18]. "Beef cattle" reach "slaughter age" by 24 months young[19]. Cattle can live 20 years or more[20]. 32,950,400 cattle were bred and slaughtered in the U.S. in 2012, – 3,151,800 of which were dairy cows[21].

*Male calves born to dairy cows have no purpose in an industry that exploits the female reproductive system, and so they are killed at anytime between 1 day young and 24 weeks young to be sold as veal[22]. 772,200 "veal calves" were bred and killed in the U.S. in 2012[23].

*Pigs can live up to 12 years[24], but they are slaughtered at 6 months young[25]. Breeding sows, who are kept to simply birth the babies who will be killed in 6 months, are killed when they are between 3 and 5 years young, after giving birth to and losing dozens of offspring[26]. 113,152,100 hogs were bred and killed in the U.S. in 2012, 3,032,400 of which were sows[27].

*Chickens bred and kept for their flesh are slaughtered around 7 weeks young[28]. Chickens bred and kept for their eggs are killed around 1 to 2 years young[29]. Chickens can live up to 8 years[30]. 8,576,161,000 chickens were bred and killed in the U.S. in 2012[31]. Chickens are classified as "poultry" a category that is not protected under the so-called Humane Slaughter Act, meaning they don't have to be stunned unconscious before having their throats cut[32].

*Turkeys are killed when they're 4 to 5 months young[33], though they have a lifespan of up to 15 years[34]. 250,192,000 turkeys were bred and killed in 2012[35]. Since turkeys are classified as "poultry" in the industry, the already poorly enforced Humane Slaughter Act doesn't apply to them, either.

*Ducks are slaughtered when they're 7 to 8 weeks young[36], though they have a lifespan of between 6 and 8 years[37]. 24,183,000 were bred and killed in 2012[38]. Since ducks are classified as "poultry" too, the "Humane Slaughter Act," doesn't protect them, either.

*Geese are slaughtered at between 15 and 20 weeks young[39]. Geese can live for between 8 and 15 years[40]. Geese were among the 121,800,000 pounds of birds, excluding chickens and turkeys, bred and slaughtered in the U.S. in 2012[41].Since they're classified as "poultry," as well, the Humane Slaughter Act does not apply to geese.

*Goats are killed between 12 and 20 weeks young[42], though they can live up to 14 years[43]. 731,800 goats were slaughtered in 2012[44].

*Rabbits are slaughtered at 10 to 12 weeks young[45], though their natural life span is 8 to 12 years[46]. Approximately 2 million[47] rabbits were killed in 2001. Since rabbits are classified as "poultry" in the industry, the "Humane Slaughter Act" doesn't apply to them, either.

*Lambs are slaughtered at 6 to 8 months young[48], though the lifespan of sheep is 12 to 14 years[49]. 2,183,000 lambs and sheep were bred and killed in the U.S. in 2012; 2,027,000 of which were lambs and yearlings.[50]

*"Squab" pigeons, sold for consumption in many U.S. restaurants, are slaughtered at 4 weeks young. The lifespan of these king pigeons is 8 to 12 years[51]. Pigeons were among the 121,800,000 pounds of birds, excluding chickens and turkeys, bred and slaughtered in the U.S. in 2012[52]. (In terms of numbers of animals, 1,294,163 pigeons were sold in the U.S. in 2007[53].)

*While horses have not been slaughtered domestically since 2007, nearly 138,000 horses were transported to Canada and Mexico in 2010 for slaughter[54]. Horses can naturally live into their 30s[55], but it is young, healthy horses who are often slaughtered[56].

HUMAN RIGHTS

Workers who labor in animal factories and slaughter-houses suffer from repetitive stress injuries as well as respiratory illnesses due to exposure to such gases as ammonia from animals' feces and urine and hydrogen sulfide from manure pits[57]. The fast line speeds, dirty killing floors, lack of training, and the struggling animals who break workers' bones, cut, and sometimes trample them, make slaughter-houses some of the most dangerous places to work in America today. What's more, those who make a living killing – on whatever size farm and for whatever purpose – become desensitized to violence – against animals and people, including loved ones. Much more work needs to be done in this area, but sociologists are beginning to document the rates of domestic abuse, alcoholism, and violent crime among slaughterhouse workers.

According to the Food Empowerment Project (food-ispower.org), a leader in raising awareness about human rights and the animal farming industry, "a large percentage of factory farm workers are people of color including migrant workers from Mexico and other parts of Latin America. An unknown percentage of full-time and part-time workers are undocumented. Employers find undocumented workers to be ideal recruits because they are less likely to complain about low wages and hazardous working conditions. Workers are largely unaware of the inherent health hazards and social struggles they will encounter in this industry. Differences in language and culture often leave workers feeling like outcasts in their new community."[58]

A WEB OF SOCIAL JUSTICE

There are still many misconceptions about vegans who "do it for the animals," and it's a joy to debunk them whenever I can. However, one that leaves me somewhat sad is the assumption that because I care about this issue – violence against animals – I don't care about other issues. That in caring about animals, I don't care about humans, as if compassion for one species means lack of compassion for another. The implication is that humans have a limited capacity for mercy, kindness, and empathy – that we don't have enough to go around.

Though I don't believe people have a limited capacity for compassion, I do think our innate childhood compassion gets dulled by the many ways in which our society seems to value convenience, pleasure, and convention above everything else. Free of the expectations imposed on us by societal mores and cultural traditions, we would discover that our hearts are large enough to hold everyone. Indeed, the more we give, the more we have to go around. What good could possibly come from parceling out our compassion in a piecemeal fashion, or creating boundaries around it? Where should those boundaries end? At different races? At different genders? At different species? Should we ration our compassion? Silly as that concept sounds, it seems to be the implication when people judge others for caring about animals.

One thing I know for sure is that problems we have in this world are not because we have so much compassion we don't know what to do with it. The problems we have in this world are because people are not living according to their *own* values of compassion and kindness. The problem is *not* the people who are doing something in this world. There are a lot of issues to address; there is a lot of work to be done, and there are millions of people doing absolutely nothing. Would that more people got up, spoke out, and did something – anything – to make this a better world for *everyone*. No, the problem is not a few people who do a lot on behalf of animals; the problem is the many people who do nothing for no one.

And the fact is, *any* work that focuses on creating non-violence and kindness in this world affects all other types of social justice. They are all connected. Compassionate people all have the same goal: the elimination of oppression, exploitation, and violence. Abuse, violence, and cruelty all spring from the same source, and they all have the same effect – more abuse, more violence, more cruelty. In his lyrically written novel, *The Unbearable Lightness of Being*, Milan Kundera writes, "Humanity's true moral test, its fundamental test, consists of its attitude toward those who are at his mercy: animals. And in this respect, human kind has suffered a fundamental debacle, a debacle so fundamental that all others stem from it."

Cesar Chavez, the late labor activist and civil rights leader – and vegetarian – also recognized that all oppressions are rooted in the same soil of violence and prejudice. He wrote, "Kindness and compassion towards all living things is a mark of a civilized society. Racism, economic deprival, dog fighting and cockfighting, bullfighting and rodeos are all cut from the same fabric: violence. Only when we have become nonviolent towards all life will we have learned to live well ourselves."[59]

Dick Gregory – author, activist, civil rights leader, and vegetarian – also recognizes this connection. He wrote, "Under the leadership of Dr. Martin Luther King, I became totally committed to nonviolence, and I was convinced that nonviolence meant opposition to killing in any form. I felt the commandment 'Thou shalt not kill' applied to human beings not only in their dealings with each other but in their practice of killing animals for food or sport. Animals and humans suffer and die alike...Violence causes the same pain, the same spilling of blood, the same stench of death, the same arrogant, cruel and brutal taking of life."

And feminist author and activist Carol Adams writes extensively about the institutionalized oppression of and violence towards women and animals. She writes that the treatment of "animals as objects" is parallel to and associated with patriarchal society's objectification of women, blacks, and other minorities in order to routinely exploit them. This paradigm is most recognizable in the exploitation of female animals for their reproductive secretions – cows for their milk that should go to their babies and hens for their eggs, which are products of their own reproductive cycles.

Whatever brings us to veganism, the benefits we experience are manifold, and they cast ripple effects far beyond what we can imagine.

CHAPTER 4:

THE JOYS AND BENEFITS
OF LIVING VEGAN

As discussed in the previous chapter, people who contemplate "becoming vegan" tend to be motivated by health, ethics, or both, and they quickly learn that – whatever the motivation – eliminating animal products from their diet reaps many benefits, some of which they've never even considered before.

One thing I can guarantee: if change is what you're looking for, then change is what you'll get, and I commend anyone who seeks it out. Change is often one of the most difficult things for humans to cope with – even when that change is positive. How many of us avoid making changes until we're absolutely forced to? How many of us engage in habits that make us sick, rather than simply change the way we eat? I've even heard doctors freely admit that they don't always give their patients the option of making significant diet changes – beyond advising them to switch from "red meat" to "white meat" – because they say people won't change.

Call me crazy, but I have more faith in people than that. I know people change. I see it every single day. When the bar is raised, and people are given the tools and resources they need to feel empowered, they *do* change. The problem is the more we keep telling people it's too hard to change, the more they just believe it.

The more we buy into the myth that there's something *radical* about eating fruits, vegetables, nuts, grains, seeds, legumes, mushrooms, herbs, and spices and that there's something *extreme* about *not* eating the mutilated bodies and stolen secretions of non-human animals, the less we'll expect of ourselves, and the less we'll expect of others. And nothing will change.

But if we hold the bar high and have some expectations, we see radical changes take place in people – physically, emotionally, and spiritually.

All I ask of people is that they remain open. Embrace the journey that encourages us to be humble, to learn new things, to become better people. That's what being human is all about: we can continually make new choices, better choices, more compassionate choices – once we know better.

Many of the changes people experience upon becoming vegan are immediate, and some are noticeable within 30 days. All of them can be broken down into several categories of positive change in terms of nutrient consumption, disease prevention and reversal, physical changes, palate sensitivity, and a sense of ethical congruency.

Nutrient Consumption Being vegan is as much about what you take in as it is about what you eliminate.

What You Can Expect None of: As soon as you eliminate meat, dairy, and eggs from your diet, I can absolutely guarantee that you will be consuming *no* dietary cholesterol, no lactose, no animal protein, no animal hormones, no animal fat, and no aberrant proteins that cause "mad cow disease" (bovine spongiform encephalopathy) – all of which originate in animal products and not in plants. Not only are these things unnecessary, they can all be harmful to the human body.

What You Can Expect More of: When you increase your consumption of plants, I can also guarantee you will be eating more fiber, more antioxidants, more folate, and more phytochemicals, because the source of these healthful substances is plants – not animals. You will also be taking in more essential vitamins and minerals, because – as you will discover below – the nutrients we need are *plant-based*.

What You Can Expect Significantly Less of: Making *whole foods* the foundation of your diet, which is what I recommend, means that you will significantly reduce your consumption of many other disease-causing substances, including:

* **Saturated Fat** – Though it exists mostly in animal flesh and secretions, saturated fat is also found in small amounts in plant foods, primarily from

coconuts. However, plant-based saturated fat is chemically different from animal-based saturated fat and does not appear to have the same negative affect on our bodies; in other words, a little virgin coconut oil, coconut butter, or coconut milk in your diet is fine – possibly even beneficial.

* **Heavy Metals** – Heavy metals such as mercury and other toxins settle in the fatty flesh of animals and are consumed by humans through their consumption of fish, dairy, and meat. The reason I didn't add this to the "Expect None" category is because even vegans consume low levels of heavy metals that end up on our food but in *significantly* less quantities.

* **Foodborne Illnesses** – Although there is still a risk of vegans consuming tainted fruits and vegetables that they buy in a store or restaurant, because they are not eating animals and their secretions, the odds of vegans contracting a foodborne illness are much lower. When you keep a vegan kitchen, the worst thing you might find is aphids in your kale and a borer worm in your corn.[60]

* **Trans Fats** – By following my recommendations for eating whole foods, you take in far fewer trans fats, which are prevalent in processed foods via partially hydrogenated oils and which are also present in animal-based meat.

Disease Prevention and Reversal

Decades of peer-reviewed research have borne out the many benefits of a vegan diet in terms of disease-prevention and reversal.

If your goal is prevention, treatment, or reversal of cardiovascular disease (particularly the atherosclerosis that causes heart attacks and strokes), you couldn't make a better dietary change than switching to a whole foods plant-based diet. And even by the end of a short period, you will see changes in the markers for these diseases – especially if you got your blood work done before you begin.

Countless studies also point to the fact that a vegan diet contributes to reduced risk of type 2 diabetes, certain cancers – particularly prostate, colon, and breast – macular degeneration, cataracts, arthritis, and osteoporosis[61].

Physical Changes

Typically, the physical changes people detect have to do with what they tend to lose, but there are gains to be made, too.

What You Can Expect to Lose: People *tend* to lose weight when they remove fat- and calorie-dense meat, dairy, and eggs from their diet because fat-laden foods have more calories than protein- and carbohydrate-rich foods. Remember: there are 4 calories per one gram of protein and one gram of carbohydrates; there are 9 calories per one gram of fat. So, when you cut out the most prevalent culprits of fat (animal products), you naturally reduce calorie intake – and thus potentially lose weight.

After a short time of eating no animal flesh or secretions, people also tend to notice a decrease in the severity of their allergies; and women tend to experience fewer PMS and menopausal symptoms.

What You Can Expect to Gain: However, it's not just what you lose – it's what you gain, too! Many people who switch to a vegan diet notice they have more energy, brighter skin with fewer blemishes, and an increase in the number of times they move their bowels, which is definitely beneficial for short- and long-term gastrointestinal health.

Palate Sensitivity

Many people report that once their palate and body begin to know life without being coated by animal-derived fat and sodium, cravings for these things are greatly reduced or totally eliminated. As a result, your palate may become more sensitive, you may taste flavors you never noticed before, and you may even have a more acute sense of smell.

Spiritual and Ethical Benefits

The harder-to-measure goals are those that have to do with what it *feels* like to make choices that reflect our values. Prior to becoming vegan, I perceived myself as a conscious, compassionate person, and yet I was supporting what is very likely the most violent industry on the planet. I was paying people to be desensitized and to do what I would never do myself: hurt and kill animals. I still consider myself a conscious, compassionate, non-violent person, but now those values are authentically reflected in my everyday behavior.

Trackable Changes

Most people find it remarkable that that the body can change and heal so quickly –with food and not pharmaceuticals, though it's been demonstrated again and again. We know this simply on an anecdotal level – feeling energized and clean after eating a healthful nutrient-dense meal or heavy and sick after a rich fat-laden meal – and this is validated on a clinical level by taking blood before and after a meal, noting differences in blood cholesterol, blood pressure, blood glucose, and the like. With our ability to measure such specifics, we know that after *one meal* our body chemistry changes negatively or positively depending on what we eat.

After *one meal*.

To be sure, the body is a complex organism, but in many ways its needs are simple. In fact, if we whittled it down, we can say that a healthy body is all about blood flow – keeping that blood flowing through our arteries to get to all the places it needs to go, easily and without hindrance.

Each time we eat, we have the choice to consume substances that hinder this blood flow or help it. After decades of research in the field of food and health, one thing is clear: animal products (meat, dairy, and eggs) *hinder* blood flow; plant foods (fruits, vegetables, grains, legumes, etc.) *increase* blood flow.

This is why people see significant, tangible, measurable changes in their blood within a few weeks of eating vegan. Like water that runs through an unblocked hose, the blood is able to run easily through the arteries – both because of the improved consistency of the blood and because of the openness of the arteries themselves.

To experience these changes, however, requires a little openness. It requires surrendering some old notions and being willing to have a new understanding. And believe me, I've heard every excuse in the book and know how attached people are to their meat and animal products.

Some people are skeptical. Having been utterly disempowered by the modern medical system, many people believe that their genes have already determined their fate, an unfortunate perspective often reinforced by their doctors. Rather than believe they have a part to play in their health, they've made scapegoats of their ancestors and simply thrown up their hands. To them I say, try eating vegan for 30 days. You have nothing to lose.

Some people say they "don't eat a lot of meat and dairy," so they think they wouldn't benefit very much from taking this stuff out of their diets completely. In the many years I've been doing this work, I've met very few people who don't have this perception of themselves. Almost every person I meet says "I don't eat a lot of meat, dairy, and eggs." But I have to ask: Compared to what? Compared to how much they *could* eat? Compared to how much they ate 100 years ago? What barometer are we using when we say that? Part of the problem is that our perception of ourselves and our habits isn't always aligned with reality. The truth is you don't know how much of this stuff you're eating until you stop, and that's one of the benefits of doing something like The 30-Day Vegan Challenge (30dayveganchallenge.com), my online program. You stop long enough to see your dietary habits very clearly. You stop long enough to realize how habitually you reach for something without thinking about it. Changing your behavior for 30 days gives you the opportunity to re-program your habits.

So to those who don't think you eat that much meat, dairy, and eggs, I say "great." It just means it will be that much easier for you to stop completely!

Some people think they're too old to make changes. Resigning themselves to the "inevitable" diseases and medications associated with "getting old," these excuse-itarians insist you can't teach an old dog new tricks. I disagree. It doesn't matter how old we are when we decide to make changes. Our food habits were ingrained in us by the time we were about 5 years old, and we carry these habits with us into adulthood. It doesn't matter if you're 30 or 40 or 18 or 80, a habit is a habit is a habit.

The behaviorists who say it takes 3 weeks to change a habit don't make qualifications based on age. They don't say it takes 3 weeks to change a habit if you're 25 years old, but 3 months to change a habit if you're 70. A habit is a habit is a habit no matter how old you are. You just have to be willing to cast off some familiar behaviors and perceptions and try on some new ones.

Although they are deeply ingrained in us, our habits do not reflect who we really are. By definition, a habit is just a behavioral pattern we've created over time. In fact, the word "habit" originally referred to something that was worn (and is still used to refer to the garb of some religious persons, such as nuns), which means it can be just as easily taken on as taken off.

That's the good news, and that's the bad news. It's the bad news because we're tenacious creatures of habit, but it's the good news because – by definition – habits can be broken.

After the initial transition period (I think 30 days is the perfect amount of time), some habits you never thought you'd be able to let go of will have fallen away effortlessly and some habits you'd never thought you'd form will become second nature. You will no doubt experience changes that are impossible to measure – changes in your outlook, energy level, perspective, and overall wellbeing – but you will also most likely experience physiological and biochemical changes that you can track and measure.

Many people get their blood and urine work done during their annual physical exam, but they tend to trust what their doctor says without ever really look at or understanding the laboratory results themselves. The guide below is meant to help you understand what the numbers mean so you can compare yours to the optimal numbers in each category. Keep in mind that common laboratory tests span a wide spectrum, so I'm including only a few. Your health professional can help you interpret others not listed here.

BODY WEIGHT

When it comes to evaluating weight and its impact on your health, it's not just a matter of what the scale says. Rather, your percentage of body fat, waist circumference, and body mass index (BMI) should all be considered.

In the last several decades, a number of different tables have been devised to help people determine their "ideal weight." The ones that were most widely used were those created by Metropolitan Life Insurance Company in 1942 and subsequently updated over the years[62].

Although on an individual basis, these height/weight tables provide very little information about an individual's health risk, they may be helpful when used in conjunction with other measurements to indicate whether or not you are within a healthy weight range.

BMI (BODY MASS INDEX)

One of the most accurate ways of assessing whether or not you are overweight or obese is to determine what percentage of your body weight is fat. However, getting accurate body fat measurements can be expensive and difficult, so the Body Mass Index (BMI) was created in 1998 by the National Institutes of Health (NIH). This guide has essentially replaced the old life insurance tables as a method to gauge healthy weight, and it helps doctors, researchers, dietitians, and government agencies get on the same page regarding weight recommendations. The same scale is used for men and for women.

BMI is a measure of body weight relative to height. Search for a BMI table online, find your height in the left-hand column, and move across the same row to the number closest to your weight. The number at the top of that column is your BMI.

According to NIH standards, you are considered over-weight if you have a BMI between 25 to 29.9 and obese if you have a BMI of 30 or higher. A healthy weight is a BMI of 18.5-24.9.[63]

One of the main problems with using the Body Mass Index *alone* is that it doesn't factor in muscle mass, so people like body builders can have a high BMI but low actual body fat. Thus, it's useful to factor in waist circumference.

WAIST CIRCUMFERENCE

Waist circumference is a helpful measurement because your health is affected not only by excess body fat, but also by *where the fat is located*. Some people gain weight in the abdominal area (the so-called "apple shape"); others, around their hips and buttocks ("pear-shaped" bodies). People with the former are at higher risk for heart disease and Type-2 diabetes.

According to the National Institutes of Health, a waist circumference greater than 40 inches for men and 35 inches for women is linked to a higher risk of Type-2 diabetes, high blood pressure, high cholesterol levels, and heart disease.[64]

To properly measure your waist, place a tape measure around your middle, just above your hipbones but below your rib cage. Breathe out, and measure.

PERCENTAGE OF BODY FAT

You can determine your body fat by using one of those little devices called calipers, often available at your local gym or doctor's office. This is basically a skinfold test to determine the thickness of the subcutaneous fat layer at three or seven sites on the body, which is then converted to estimate fat percentage. According to the American Council on Exercise, a body fat level greater than 17% in men and 27% in women indicates one is overweight, while a body fat level of more than 25% in men and 31% in women indicates obesity.[65]

BLOOD PRESSURE

Blood pressure is a measure of how hard blood is pressing against artery walls, like water running through a hose. Ideally, you want the top number to be under 120 and the bottom number under 80. The risk for strokes and heart attacks starts progressively climbing after 115/75 mmHg. You can test your blood pressure using machines available in many pharmacies and doctor's offices, or buy a device to check at home. See Recommended Resources at the end of the book.[66]

BLOOD GLUCOSE

According to the American Diabetes Association, it is estimated that 18.8 million people (children and adults) in the United States have been diagnosed with diabetes, another 7 million are undiagnosed, and 79 million are pre-diabetic.[67]

One to three different glucose tests are given by doctors to make a diagnosis.

* The first test checks the amount of glucose in your blood at any given time during the day, regardless of the last meal eaten. A glucose value of 200 mg/dl (plus diabetes symptoms) is a good indicator of diabetes.

* The second test is a fasting blood glucose, which is done after you have fasted for at minimum eight hours. Fasting glucose should be in the range of 70 to 110 mg/dl; a fasting glucose level of 126 mg/dl or more indicates diabetes.

* The third test is an oral glucose tolerance test to see how well your body deals with sugar. Normally, blood sugar rises after you eat and then returns to normal levels (70 to 110 mg/dl) within an hour or two. Higher values means your body has trouble moving glucose out of the blood and into the cells.

The 79 million people with "pre-diabetes" means their fasting blood glucose level is 110 to 125 and post-meal level is 140 to 200 mg/dl – not high enough to be considered diabetes but higher than what is considered normal[68].

CHOLESTEROL

When it comes to talking about cholesterol, we throw around labels such as "good" and "bad," though many of us don't even know what cholesterol is or what it does. Made in the liver of animals, cholesterol is a fat-like substance we consume in our diets via meat, dairy, and eggs (there is no dietary cholesterol in plant foods). Though our bodies also produce cholesterol (we are, after all, animals), we have no requirement to *consume* dietary cholesterol. The cholesterol made by our bodies travels through the bloodstream in little packages called *lipoproteins*:

* Low-density lipoproteins (LDL or "bad" cholesterol) deliver cholesterol TO the body.

* High-density lipoproteins (HDL or "good" cholesterol) take cholesterol OUT of the bloodstream.

When there is too much cholesterol in the bloodstream, it's a major risk factor for heart and blood vessel disease. To determine cardiovascular disease risk, doctors look at total cholesterol, LDL, HDL, and the ratio of the latter two.

Total Cholesterol: Because the average cholesterol level in the United States is so high (around 200[69]), recommendations indicate that levels must be reduced to "below 200." Although it's true that people with a level of 200 are at lower risk than those at 235, they are still at significantly high risk. In fact, about 35% of those who have heart attacks have cholesterol levels between 160 and 200.[70]

After decades of research, including longtime landmark studies such as the Framingham Heart Study and the China Diet Study, it is evident that the optimal level for total cholesterol is below 150. What's more, those with a cholesterol level under 150 don't really have to concern themselves with the further breakdown of "good" and "bad" cholesterol analysis, outlined below.

LDL ("Bad") Cholesterol: Less than 100 is the optimal number.

HDL ("Good") Cholesterol: Between 40 and 60 is optimal.

Important Note: A nutrient-dense plant-based diet makes the HDL portion of cholesterol *lower* because *all* portions of the *total cholesterol* are reduced. In other words, don't think something is wrong when your HDL level falls. On the other hand, a very high HDL level (60 or above) is not always a good sign either. It means the HDL is working harder to get cholesterol out of the bloodstream. The more cholesterol, the more work it has to do.

TRIGLYCERIDES

Triglycerides are fatty substances that – like cholesterol – are made in the liver and circulate in the bloodstream. High levels indicate a risk of cardiovascular disease and are associated with pancreatitis.

Although medical establishments consider triglyceride levels of 100 to 150 mg/dL "normal" or "good," many experts feel that optimal fasting blood triglyceride levels should be 50 to 150 milligrams mg/dL). Levels of 200 to 500 mg/dL are considered high and very high, respectively.[71]

HOMOCYSTEINE

Homocysteine is an amino acid that is normally found in small amounts in the blood. Higher levels are associated with increased risk of cardiovascular disease, venous thrombosis, dementia, and Alzheimer's disease.

The optimal range is between 6 and 8 μmol/L.[72]

Helpful Note: Keeping homocysteine at levels associated with lower rates of disease requires both adequate intake of vitamin B12 (through supplements or fortified foods) and folate (through green leafy vegetables) or folic acid (the synthetic version of folate found as single supplements or in multivitamins).

VITAMINS

Because there are some vitamin deficiencies in the typical American diet, it is also worth looking at the following:

* **Vitamin D** – Americans are deficient in vitamin D more any other vitamin. Experts' opinions vary between shooting for 40 to 60 ng/mL and 50 to 70 ng/mL as the optimal range.[73]

* **B12**: >400 pg/mL is optimal. (In the case of getting an accurate B12 level checked, it's recommended that you request a urine MMA test or get it online. See Recommended Resources at the end of the book.[74]

Dealing with Changes

I've had the privilege and honor of ushering thousands of people through the vegan transition, and I know that even as they feel more grounded, more energetic, and more joyful, they are often quite overwhelmed by how profound these transformations are. Some changes people experience are purely physiological, both the macro changes that take place in terms of cholesterol, blood pressure, blood glucose, etc. and also visible changes – changes you can feel and see. Other changes are less tangible.

PHYSICAL CHANGES

Coping with Fiber: Because there is no fiber in meat, dairy, eggs, or any animal product, many people are eating a very low-fiber diet. When you initially increase your intake of plant foods – and thus fiber – you may experience some discomfort. However, once your body adjusts, it's not really a problem for most people. In the beginning, if you feel you need to take in fewer high-fiber foods, you can still do so without adding animal products back into your diet. There are lower-fiber plant foods you can try, such as white rice instead of brown, bagels, pastas, crackers, tofu, non-dairy yogurt, tomato sauce, pizza, fruit juices (with no pulp), apple sauce, and bananas. As you get more comfortable – and you will – you can continue adding more fiber-rich plant foods into your diet.

The Power of Fiber: Unlike the soluble fiber that helps to reduce cholesterol and stabilize blood sugar, insoluble fiber is the plant roughage that stays in tact and helps push everything through and out of our bodies, manifesting in more trips to the bathroom. Some people get nervous about this; but it's not only normal, it's optimal. The average non-vegan has sub-optimal fiber intake, which contributes to less-frequent bowel movements and constipation, marked by hard, dry, hard-to-pass stools. So, even though you may be surprised by the new sensations in your colon or by the change in your stool from hard pellets to a softer final product, you can celebrate the fact that this is quite literally contributing to reduced risk of colon disease and cancer.

Discomforting Beans: It's the sugar molecules – called oligosaccharides – in beans that people have a hard time digesting, resulting in gas, cramping, or bloating. Rather than avoiding eating these healthful legumes, there are a number of things you can do if beans give you trouble.

* Gradually increase your intake of beans. Counter-intuitive though it may seem, the more your body becomes adjusted to these oligosaccharides, the easier it is for it to digest them. Throw a few on a salad or into a soup, and slowly begin to eat more concentrated bean dishes.

* Eat more canned beans than beans made from scratch. In canned beans, the sugars have been aggressively cooked out, and the beans have been rinsed really well, making these oligosaccharides less prevalent.

* If you cook beans from scratch, *do not* cook the beans in the same water you soaked them in. Also, try adding kombu seaweed to the beans while they're cooking, or add a little white vinegar to the beans just after they're cooked.

* People tend to do better with the smaller lentils than with the larger beans. Give that a try and see if it helps.

* Some species of a particular mold produce an anti-oligosaccharide enzyme, which facilitates digestion of oligosaccharides in the small intestine. This enzyme is currently sold in the U.S. under the brand-name *Beano*. By taking this enzyme at the same time you begin to eat the beans, there's a very good chance that you won't experience the gas and bloating. However, the only problem with Beano is that it uses gelatin to make its capsule. Fret not. A vegan version called *Bean-zyme* is available in health food stores, large natural grocery stores, and online stores.

Reduced Pre-Menstrual Symptoms: Hormones thrive on fat, so when you reduce your consumption of dietary fat – which happens naturally when you eliminate meat, dairy, and eggs – you may find that you have a shorter menstrual period, less bleeding, less cramping, and a more regular cycle. Women going through menopause may also experience fewer symptoms, and post-menopausal women may find they no longer need synthetic hormones (check with your doctor). To be sure, these are all positive changes, but they're worth mentioning here in case you've noticed these changes and were wondering if they were normal.

Cravings: When we eliminate animal flesh and secretions from our diet and experience what we call "physical cravings," we are most likely craving fat and salt. Just as with any substance we have been habitually putting in our bodies, we will no doubt go through some withdrawals when it's removed. After some time has passed, your body and palate will have altered enough that you stop craving the heavy, fat- and salt-laden foods you once ate with abandon.

The Vegan Glow: When you eat a large amount of beta-carotene-rich foods, you may notice your skin begin to take on an orange glow. There is nothing wrong with this. However, if you want to tone down the tint, you can still eat carotenoid-rich foods that aren't orange. (To put it in perspective: one medium carrot contains 330% of your daily value of vitamin A; one cup of raw spinach contains 75%.)

There is another glow I've seen in many vegans, which is the light that emanates from within in. Many talk about a sense of peace and calm that comes from aligning their values with their behavior, and it shines through their skin and their eyes. This is obviously not a problem to solve. Embrace it.

EMOTIONAL CHANGES

Guilt: I've heard from a number of people who experience feelings of guilt after they stop eating animals and their milk and eggs. Lucidly aware of how they once contributed to animal suffering, they are now trying to cope with that awareness and seek to make symbolic amends to the animals they once ate. They can do this by contributing to vegan and farmed animal organizations, and by visiting farmed animal sanctuaries and bonding with individual animals who serve as ambassadors for their respective species. The most helpful remedy for dealing with the past is creating a better future, and the best way to do this is by being part of the solution. Not eating animals, being a joyful advocate for veganism, and speaking up for the voiceless are all significant ways to accomplish this.

Anger: The stereotype of the angry vegan is well known, and though it is indeed a stereotype, there is no doubt that people feel anger once they learn about the heinous abuses committed against animals. And whereas many people feel a sense of peace at no longer participating in and paying for these abuses to take place, the awareness of so much cruelty and suffering can also have a devastating effect on our psyches, and the result is sometimes anger.

And why shouldn't people be angry? Human greed and the desire for convenience and pleasure drive the socially sanctioned use and abuse of billions of nonhuman animals. We live in a world where it's considered normal to champion this and radical to oppose it. Of course people are angry. But anger is not a dirty word. It is a very real response, whose roots go deep. It's what we do with anger that will make or break us.

I think it's very helpful to know that the root of the word *anger* is *sorrow* or *anguish*. The earliest roots of the word *anger* referred to something being "painfully constricted," a "strangling, narrowing, squeezing, throttling." And it's anguish that people feel when we learn what happens to animals. If we reframe anger so we see it in its proper context, we can recognize that there isn't a contradiction between the peace that comes with eating nonviolently and the anger we feel in the face of so much cruelty. The key is transforming anger into action. It's easy to become cynical, disheartened and hopeless, but that doesn't do anyone any good. The key is in becoming active and staying hopeful.

Change: Even when it's incredibly positive, change is still change, and many people find it very difficult to deal with. There's a reason we're so habit-oriented. We feel comforted by our routines and habitual choices. They add order and familiarity to our lives, which is why some people resist change – even when it can save their lives. In fact, our society is set up to *discourage* change. Instead of being taught to change poor habits, we're given band-aids to simply cover them up; we romanticize, ritualize, and justify harmful behavior just so we don't have to do anything about it.

Hopefully, once you realize that change is not so scary, you will feel empowered to continue. You start exercising muscles you never knew you had, and you begin to know yourself a little better. That alone is a reward, even though there is so much more.

CHAPTER 5:

READING LABELS

Contrary to what many people think, vegans do not spend all their time deciphering labels. Once you know what to look for, one quick glance at the label will tell you whether something has an animal product in it. Having said that, if you have to weed through a long list of ingredients to determine if it's vegan or not, you probably shouldn't be eating that product anyway. Why would you want to eat something that resembles a chemistry experiment rather than actual food? You shouldn't feel like you're in science class when you read a label.

The best way to avoid labels altogether is to eat whole foods as much as possible. The more you eat whole foods, the less you have to worry about animal products or unnecessary and potentially harmful ingredients in your food.

However, I don't think it's realistic to expect people to eat nothing but whole fruits, whole vegetables, and whole grains. Although making these foods the *foundation* of our diet is what I recommend, it's helpful to know what to look for when we're buying perfectly healthful things such as canned beans, premade soups, packaged tortillas, premade tomato sauce, condiments, and the like.

When reading labels, I recommend choosing:

* foods with the fewest ingredients possible (making exceptions, of course, when something includes a number of spices and herbs)

* ingredients with recognizable names

* ingredients that are animal-free

Now, some people argue that once you eliminate the most obvious animal products from your diet (meat, animal's milk, and eggs), you can relax a bit when it comes to the animal products hidden in commercial foods. Although being vegan is not about obsessing over being perfect, I simply don't want to consume the blood, bones, or fat of animals – even when they're hidden among other ingredients. I would never buy any of these things if they were sold individually, and I don't want to eat them shoved into my food as filler or fat. In fact, many of these animal products are given names other than what they really are because even the manufacturers know that people wouldn't buy them if they knew exactly what they were.

Look out for the following:

Gelatin: Made by boiling the remaining bones, skin, and connective tissues of slaughtered animals – most often cattle, pigs, horses, and fishes – gelatin is the by-product of the meat and leather industries. If it says "gelatin" on the label, it is from an animal. Though there are vegetable-derived "gelatins" available, particularly in the form of agar, guar gum, carrageenan, and pectin, they are NOT the source if a label simply says "gelatin."

* Products most associated with gelatin are Jell-O, marshmallows, vitamin capsules, gummy bears, and ice cream. Vegan versions of each are available.

* **ETHICAL CONSIDERATION**: Though gelatin is made from the "by-products" of slaughterhouse waste, it is misguided to think that using the remains of the animals is a noble use of what would "go to waste," as many people assert. We unnecessarily kill 10 billion land animals and countless marine animals every year, and the industries who profit off of these animals have come up with sundry ways to make even more money by selling their byproducts. These very profitable byproduct industries simply wouldn't exist if we didn't systematically kill animals in the first place. By purchasing animal byproducts, we are supporting the primary industries we ethically oppose.

Whey and casein: Both are both derived from animal's milk. When you curdle dairy-based milk (to make cheese), you are essentially separating the milk solids (casein) from the milk liquid (whey). If the label says "casein," "casein-ate," "milk protein," "sodium caseinate," or "whey," these ingredients are most definitely animal-derived. Some soy- and rice-based cheeses contain casein.

* Products most associated with casein and whey: Some - but not all - brands of protein powders, boxed cereals, cereal bars, processed sandwich breads, prepared bread crumbs, and crackers contain these cow's milk derivatives. Vegan versions of these foods are definitely available, so just check the label.

* **HEALTH CONSIDERATION**: When you separate the curds from the whey to make cheese, you're tangling up all the milk proteins (the casein) into solid masses or "curds." What remains contains only whey proteins. In cow's milk, 80%-87% of the proteins are caseins, which is not a good thing. According to renowned researcher and Professor Emeritus of Nutritional Biochemistry at Cornell University, T. Colin Campbell, casein is the "number one carcinogen (i.e. cancer-causing substance) that people come in contact with on a daily basis." In dairy-based cheeses, the casein is even more concentrated, and in low-fat dairy-based milks, there tends to be more casein to make up for the fat that has been removed.

Lactose: The sugar in all mammalian milk (including humans), lactose appears on labels as such. However, "lactate" or "lactic acid" is not animal-derived.

* **HEALTH CONSIDERATION**: There seems to be a misunderstanding about the components that make up mammalian milk, since I often hear people mistakenly assert that they're "allergic to milk" and thus drink lactose-free cow's milk. Casein is the milk protein to which people can become allergic; lactose is the milk sugar that gives many people gas, bloating, and cramps. Since so many people are suffering from "lactose intolerance," which is our body's natural revulsion to a sugar we're not equipped to digest after we're weaned, the dairy industry came up with a profitable solution: lactose-free milk. Though the milk may not contain lactose, it still contains saturated fat, dietary cholesterol, and casein. If you want truly lactose-free milk, drink those derived from plants.

Lanolin: A fat derived from sheep's wool, lanolin is a by-product of the wool industry, and it is most commonly found in cosmetics, lotions, moisturizers, and lip balms. The Procter & Gamble product "Oil of Olay" is derived from the word "lanolin," which is a primary ingredient. (When contacted, the company confirmed that only their body washes do not contain lanolin.) Plenty of beauty products are made without lanolin.

Stearate or Stearic Acid: A fat derived from either plant or animal sources, it's used for making candles, soaps, and plastics; it's sometimes used in chewing gum and candy. The best way to know its source is to read the label. If it's plant-derived, it will most likely say so.

Carmine or Cochineal: Both of these terms refer to the ground-up bodies of beetles that are then used as a coloring in red-color juices, dairy-based yogurt and ice cream, and cosmetics. The word carmine is derived from a word that means "crimson," so essentially you'll find it in products that are some shade of red, pink, or purple. It also appears on labels as "carminic acid."

Bonito are dried fish flakes frequently seen in Japanese foods.

Lard is the fat taken from pigs' stomachs. Many Mexican restaurants make their refried beans without lard and use vegetable-based oils, instead. Just ask.

Lipoids or Lipids are the fat and fat-like substances found in animals and plants. When they're from plants, the label usually says so.

Rennet or Rennin is an enzyme taken from the fourth stomach of young ruminants to make dairy-based cheese. Each ruminant produces the special kind of rennet needed to digest his or her mother's milk. There's kid-goat rennet especially for goat's milk cheese, lamb-rennet for sheep's-milk cheese, and calf rennet for cow's milk cheese. In the case of the latter, most of the stomachs are from the discarded males of the dairy industry who are sold to the veal industry.

Isinglass is derived from the bladders of sturgeon fish and used as a clarifying agent in some wines, though it's not in the final product. Any wine labeled "vegan" means that it wasn't clarified with isinglass.

Aside from learning to recognize these animal products, another way to tell if a product is vegan is to look for the Vegan-Certified logo. Administered by an organization called Vegan Action (vegan.org), you'll find this symbol on food, clothing, cosmetics and other items that contain no animal products and are not tested on animals.

WARNING LABELS

These days we also see a lot of warnings on labels that say the food was manufactured in plants and on equipment that have also been used for cow's milk and other allergens. This is more about liability protection than anything else. The Food Allergy Labeling and Consumer Protection Act now requires labeling of any food that contains or was in contact with machinery that saw one or more of the following allergens: peanuts, soybeans, cow's milk, eggs, fish, crustacean shellfish, tree nuts, and wheat.

People have asked me if I – from a vegan perspective – buy or eat products that may be processed using machinery that also has non-vegan products processed on them. My answer is: yes I do. That kind of low-level concern about purity is not why I'm vegan, and it doesn't mean I'm less vegan if I eat chocolate chips that were processed on machinery that may also process non-vegan chips.

Being vegan is about doing the best we can in this imperfect world. It's not about being perfect or pure. If we lose sight of that, if we treat veganism as the end rather than the means, then we'll not only drive ourselves crazy, we'll also forget what being vegan is all about. Though there are some things we have no control over, I think it makes more sense to focus on what we can do rather than on what we can't.

And there's so much we can do.

CHAPTER 6:

DRAWING THE LINE – HOW VEGAN IS VEGAN?

Although I've said this before, it's worth saying again: being vegan is about doing what we can to foster compassion and to avoid contributing to violence. I believe that people genuinely do not want to contribute to animal abuse, and I also believe that it's human nature to try and take the easy way out of something, especially if it looks like there is one. When it comes to consuming animal flesh and fluids, people tend to want to have their meat (or eggs or dairy) and eat it, too. In other words, if people think they can continue eating the way they always have without being *too* inconvenienced and still feel good about all the choices they make, they'd probably consider that an ideal scenario. And they seem to have found it in the labeling of animal products.

I believe that one of the reasons we're in such a sorry state in terms of our relationship with animals is because we view them as objects for us to do with as we please. We see their flesh, skin, reproductive outputs (milk and eggs), fur, hair, bodies as here for us to use, abuse, and consume. Of course there are natural cycles we all benefit from (bees pollinating trees enabling us to eat nuts and fruit, for instance), but that need not include taking everything animals produce and commodifying them for our pleasure and profit.

Happy Chickens' Eggs

Most people immediately recognize the ethical problems with animal factories and the products that come out of them, such as chicken's eggs. To distance themselves from this obvious and inherent cruelty, they declare that they buy and eat only "free-range," "organic," and "cage-free" eggs, eggs from a neighbor's chickens, from Farmer Joe's hens down the road, or from their own "backyard chickens." I discuss the deception of the "free-range/cage-free" label elsewhere in my work, including in my podcast, but for now, I want to focus on what some people see as a genuine dilemma: "If someone has their own hens and takes excellent care of them until they die naturally, what's wrong with eating their eggs?"

First and foremost, eggs are neither healthful nor necessary in the human diet. They're loaded with cholesterol, animal fat, and potentially harmful animal protein, and whatever few nutrients they do provide are there because chickens eat plants (or have their feed laced with plant-based supplements). Instead of going *through* non-human animals to get to the nutrients we need, we need to skip the "middle animal" and go directly to the source – directly to the plants where the nutrients reside. So, I simply cannot advocate the consumption of chicken's eggs – or any bird's eggs, for that matter.

But in terms of *ethics* and not health, it seems pretty innocuous, right? After all, hens are females, and as a natural part of a female's reproductive system, eggs are secreted out of the body, whether they're fertilized or unfertilized (unlike with humans, where only unfertilized eggs are secreted out of the body through menstruation). A fertilized egg will bring forth a new chick, though an unfertilized egg will not. If there is no rooster, there is no chance the hens' eggs will become fertilized. No male, no fertilized egg, no chick, so it's not as if you're eating the unborn – just the gelatinous membranes that create the conditions for a chick to develop. This entire egg-production process happens without any human intervention or manipulation, and the hens can proceed while living out their lives in as natural a setting as possible, where they can roam in the grass, perch in the trees, bask in the sun, bathe in the dust, and do all the things chickens naturally do. So what could possibly be unethical about eating their eggs?

On the outset, it's true that there appears to be no exploitation, cruelty, or harm, but one need only scratch beneath the surface to unearth the ethical considerations, and I suggest that they have to do with *intention* behind the keeping of the hens.

Ethical Considerations

There is a very different mindset when you view an animal as a "companion" than when you view her as a "commodity." A local farmer or a backyard hobbyist who keeps hens in order to sell or eat their eggs has very different motivations and will make very different decisions than someone who has the means and desire to care for hens for the hens' own sake. Someone who adopts hens as companion animals is focused on the animals' needs – not on what the hens "produce." It's the difference between perceiving the intrinsic value of the animals versus perceiving the animals as valuable because of the benefit they bring to humans. It may seem like a subtle difference, but in fact, the consequences of such a distinction are profound.

Just because someone cares about the hens they keep for eggs doesn't mean he wouldn't kill them or sell them to be killed when they're no longer "useful" – when their production wanes to such a degree that it costs more to care for them relative to the profit gained by selling their eggs. Killing unproductive and underproductive hens is done by people who label their eggs "humane," "free-range," and "cage-free." It's done by people who declare their hens "happy," and it's done on farms called "local," "sustainable," or "organic."

The fact is there is no such thing as a slaughter-free animal agricultural system. Even sweet Farmer Joe, who sells his hens' eggs at the local farmer's market, lives by this principle – however nice a person he may be. He might call it the "harsh reality" of farming, as if it's inevitable and he has no choice. And though it's true that it is harsh – bringing someone into this world only to use her up until she's no longer valuable, then killing her – it's not true that we have no choice. We *do* have a choice. Whenever we purchase eggs – from a major supplier or from a local farm, we are perpetuating a violent cycle and subscribing to a system that views animals as products. Consuming animals – and their milk or eggs – is neither necessary nor inevitable.

Okay, you say, what about the individual who buys a couple of hens in order to eat the eggs themselves? They're not selling the eggs, they've fallen in love with their "ladies," and they'll never sell them to be slaughtered or kill them themselves. What about the ethics around eating *their* eggs?

To explore this scenario, we have to look not at the *killing* of the hens once they're underproductive but the *hatching* of the hens. In order to have hens who lay eggs for consumers to eat, they have to come from somewhere – they have to be bred. The majority of hens used for egg production purposes – on small farms or large – are bred in hatcheries. Breeder hens are inseminated so they lay *fertile* eggs ready to bring forth chicks who will then supply the egg industry. The fertile eggs are placed in incubators and, approximately 21 days later[75], thousands of beautiful chicks use their "egg teeth" to break their way out of their protective shell.

As a matter of course, within 72 hours, these babies are "sexed" by people to determine who is male and who is female[76]. Females are de-beaked and sometimes de-toed (though the industry prefers the innocuous-sounding "beak-trimming" and "toe-clipping," calling to mind a pleasant day at the spa rather than the painful procedures they are), then sold to the egg industry, where they are caged, confined, and manipulated to produce as many eggs as possible in their short lives[77]. According to the USDA, a hen kept for egg production lays an egg about once every 25 hours[78]. Laying up to 300 eggs over the course of a year is grotesquely higher than the number of eggs laid by feral chickens or breeds that closely resemble wild jungle fowl[79]. First of all, wild birds don't naturally lay eggs year-round, as production hens are forced to, and the most number of eggs that even a very productive, broody hen could conceivably lay in a spring/summer cycle would be 60 eggs a year[80].

With the calcium stripped from their bones in order for their bodies to produce shell after shell for her eggs, she is brittle-boned and cage-weary by the time she is sent to slaughter to become chicken soup or pot pie.

Back at the hatcheries – large and small – if the newly hatched chick is male (hence, a rooster), having no value in an industry that exploits the female reproductive system, he is killed through one of several methods: suffocation, maceration, electrocution, cervical dislocation, or carbon dioxide poisoning[81]. Between 470 and 490 million chickens are hatched for the egg industry each year, half of which are male[82]. Taking into account a 3-5% mortality rate in the first 10 days of their lives, that leaves approximately 230 million male rooster chicks who are killed at hatcheries every year in the United States[83]. Operations that sell "free-range" or "cage-free" eggs purchase their "layers" from these hatcheries, and there are even smaller hatcheries (breeding and hatching about 20 million chicks per year, half of whom are male[84]) that cater to "backyard chicken enthusiasts," who use the chickens for their eggs or kill them for their flesh. Some hatcheries even admit to using the unwanted male chicks as "packing peanuts."

So, is there something ethically problematic with buying hens to keep them for their eggs, even while caring for her and never killing her? If these hens were born in a hatchery where male chicks are killed and females sold to the egg industry, then I would certainly say so. Purchasing those hens perpetuates the cycle of doomed births, pain-ridden lives, and premature and gruesome deaths.

However, in the instance I described above in which the hens are adopted from a farmed animal sanctuary, they are kept as pets and will not be killed, and the people will buy no more hens, then technically speaking, there appears to be no harm in eating their eggs, if one chooses to do so.

But, this is an *extremely rare* exception. Most people are unaware that they're even purchasing hens whose lives began in hatcheries, and if they choose to never buy a hen again after learning this, it's only because they can afford to. In other words, they're individuals who are not in the business of selling eggs. Those who sell eggs for profit – even if it's an auxiliary arm of their primary crop sales – perpetuate the hatchery-slaughter cycle. But this is not how it's marketed to the public.

No one in the business of selling animal products wants to advertise the violence inherent in farming animals for their flesh, hair, fur, or secretions. You will never see printed on an egg carton label: "Hens purchased from a hatchery that macerates male chicks at birth" or "at end of their 'production cycle,' all egg-laying hens are killed by knife wounds while fighting for their lives." Every purveyor of meat, dairy, and eggs wants the public to perceive their products as humane and healthy. So, while I encourage you to inquire about the living conditions of the hens whose eggs you eat, I guarantee that unless you probe, Farmer Joe will not tell you about these hidden realities.

When visiting (or calling) a local farm or farm stand, you might ask:

> ***From where were the hens originally purchased?** Whether they say they breed them themselves or purchase them from hatcheries, ask what happens to the males. If they say they don't know what happens to the males at the hatcheries they purchase the hens from, ask for the name of the hatcheries so you can inquire yourself (and perhaps even inform the farmer so he knows what he's contributing to, assuming he doesn't).

> ***What happens to the hens when their egg-laying slows down?** Is the farmer going to pay for the care and feeding of the animals who don't provide any income in return? It's a poor business model indeed to spend money without getting a return

on your investment. Farmers are not in business as philanthropists, but the way some people romanticize animal agriculture, you'd think animal farms were sanctuaries and farmers were animal advocates.

*When the hens are sick, are they taken to the vet to receive medication and treatment? What about their convalescence? Are there special barns where sick or dying hens are kept or humanely euthanized? Again, good businesses strike a balance between profit and loss; when the latter exceeds the former, you have a failing business. Investing dollars into ailing animals or into administering proper euthanasia contributes to loss – not profit – and is simply unsound business practices. If the animals are not serving their purpose – producing to increase profits – then they're simply expendable. It's really that simple.

Egg-Eating Vegans?

Do some people truly care about their hens and treat them as part of the family? Absolutely! Will some of these farmers care for the hens their entire lives, providing them with medical care, shelter, and food until they die a natural death? Sure – a select few might be spared and kept as "pets." Will some people consider these chickens just possessions to help them make a buck and "replace" them when they get older and their egg production naturally wanes? Absolutely! Will they sell them to slaughter to get new hens? No doubt! Will they kill the hens themselves in order to get younger chickens? Inevitably!

And therein lies the difference between having hens as companions and keeping hens in order to eat their eggs. The former is often the case when vegans adopt hens from animal sanctuaries, an ideal scenario where the chickens will live out their lives in a loving home and the sanctuary frees up space and money to rescue more animals. Most farmed animal sanctuaries have strict adoption policies, whereby the adopters agree never to sell, breed, or kill the animals they adopt, and the sanctuaries are committed to taking the animals back if the people can no longer care for them.

So this begs the question, then: "If someone is vegan in every other way, but they eat the eggs of their beloved companion hens/rescued hens, is that unethical and is that person still vegan?"

It's not for me to judge if someone is "truly vegan" or not, but for all intents and purposes, one of the primary things that characterizes being vegan is that you don't consume animals and their secretions. But, that's not an arbitrary rule that exists for its own sake. The way I see it, being vegan is not an *end*; it's a *means* to an end, and to me, that end is unconditional compassion. If we get wrapped up in the *label*, we're treating veganism as the *end* – not the *means* to compassion. What I'm most interested in is changing the existing paradigm from one that sees animals as subjects of ours to use to a paradigm that treats them as co-habitants, as fellow earthlings with whom we share the planet. Because we currently see animals as here for us to do with as we please, we perceive their bodies and reproductive outputs as ours to take. We need to change our position from one of entitlement to one of communality.

In other words, chickens don't lay eggs because humans have figured out that they can act as binders for baked goods. Hens don't lay eggs – for *me*. Hens are not here – *for me*. Their eggs are not *mine*. I'd just as soon leave them alone.

For someone who identifies as vegan, who has adopted sanctuary hens and has contemplated eating their eggs, I might suggest that one possible outcome of eating their eggs is that it will keep you tied to (or return you to) old habits – and thus the paradigm of entitlement. You would still have – or you might redevelop – a penchant for the taste and habit of eating chicken's eggs, which means not only would your consumption of them displace more healthful foods in your diet, but you may continue to use – or begin to use again – chicken's eggs in your cooking and baking, leaving you tethered to old habits and unexposed to new ones.

I also think that for some people it could potentially create a slippery slope, where it becomes easier to justify eating chicken's eggs in other circumstances, reasoning that it wouldn't hurt to have eggs *just this one time* at that restaurant or at this person's house. It's possible – certainly not a guarantee – that continuing to eat chicken's eggs from rescued hens means we keep one foot in a non-vegan paradigm, making it easier to make non-vegan choices at other times in our daily lives. It's just a precaution worth considering.

The only other reason I'd be concerned about "vegans eating the eggs of their hens" is from a public relations perspective. Veganism is undermined, negated, derided, and misunderstood by so many people and in the media, and I think it confuses the public when a vegan declares they eat any animal products at all. And because the public tends to thrive on and hear only sound bites, there often isn't the opportunity to explain in 7 seconds the nuanced realities about what typically happens to chickens from cradle to grave. In other words, it doesn't help to shift the paradigm.

For anyone who cares for hens as companions and doesn't eat their eggs, the eggs don't necessarily have to go to waste. Spending as much time at farmed animal sanctuaries as I have, I've seen many of them collect the eggs, hard-boil them, then mash them up – shell and all – and feed them back to the hens to eat. The hens love them. Although it's not unheard of for birds to sometimes eat their own (obviously raw) eggs in the wild, it can create a bit of a mess, so best not to let them get a taste of the raw eggs, lest they form a habit and cannibalize their eggs before you've had a chance to retrieve them. Of course, you can also give the hard-boiled (not raw!) eggs to your other companion animals, such as your dogs or cats.

The romanticizing of animal agriculture and the increasing popularity of keeping "backyard hens" raises many troubling concerns for me, and I talk about this in greater detail elsewhere in my work, but an important issue to consider in the context of this particular chapter is the perception by some that the solution to the inevitable killing of "spent hens" (hens who no longer produce enough eggs to justify their lives) is to give them to animal sanctuaries once they're no longer wanted or "useful." I've even heard some people say this is the perfect close-loop system: hens are cared for while their egg production is high, then instead of killing them, they can be given to sanctuaries where they live out their lives in peace.

This is far from a workable solution. Farmed animal sanctuaries exist as nonprofit organizations in order to rescue and care for abused, neglected, and abandoned victims of the animal exploitation industries. It is not the mission of animal sanctuaries to support backyard chicken hobbyists or animal farmers – large or small – and none of them have the means to do so. If we truly want a closed-loop system, we would stop breeding animals for the purpose of using and killing them. Truly closing the loop requires that we change the paradigm and let go of some of our unnecessary, wasteful, and unhealthful habits – however old they may be.

Milk-"Giving" Cows, Goats, and Sheep

Similar to the chicken question, some people ask, "What's wrong with having your own dairy goat or cow if she's treated like one of the family?" My answer to this question is much less nuanced than my answer to the egg question. In fact, it's pretty clear-cut: unlike birds who happen to lay eggs as part of their reproductive cycle, mammals' bodies *have* to be manipulated in order to produce the milk humans take, inevitably destroying lives in the process.

I remember the day I learned that cows don't just naturally "give milk." I was well into my adulthood, and I remember feeling really stupid. I was an intelligent person. I understood the fundamentals of biology. And yet, because I hadn't been encouraged to think otherwise, I had completely wiped out of my mind that in order for cows to lactate, being the mammals they are, they have to be pregnant – hence the shared root word in *mammal* and *mammary*: having to do with the milk-producing glands. I believed the story I was sold because I desperately didn't want to believe that my consumption of cow's milk, cheese, and butter was harming anyone.

Prior to this realization, I had believed that cows were somehow biologically designed to bestow upon humans the gifts of their mammary glands. Even our language perpetuates this belief: we don't "take" milk; cows "give" milk – a romanticized depiction of what is nothing less than an exploitative process creating much misery and sorrow.

In order to induce cows to lactate (to produce milk), cows *must* be impregnated. In order to keep them lactating to keep the milk production high (and the cows worth keeping alive), they *must* be impregnated again and again. Cows gestation period is 9 months – almost as long as a human's. At the end of that time, when she gives birth, all she wants is her baby – just like a human.

Instead of being able to tend to her offspring, however, the dairy cow's baby is taken from her within days (sometimes a day) of birth, a process that every dairy producer – of either a large or small operation – will admit is incredibly stressful for both mother and baby. Fiercely protective, a mother cow will do anything to keep her offspring safe and by her side, but it's a fight she never wins. In the end, her calf is taken from her, and she spends days brooding and bellowing – before being impregnated again. Her milk is taken from her almost the entire time she is pregnant; most operations provide her with a 60-day "dry-off" period, where they stop milking her 60 days before giving birth, but many push it to 45 days, which is extremely stressful on the cow[85].

It's important to keep in mind that the offspring of a dairy cow (or goat or sheep) is merely incidental. He or she exists only because a cow (or doe or ewe) needs to be made pregnant in order to lactate. The dairy industry is all about stimulating and increasing milk production, and the offspring is just the undesired consequence of a forced pregnancy. And because the dairy industry is just that – a profit-driven business – the decisions made about the fate of the animals are dictated by motivations for profit – not compassion.

If the offspring is a female, she becomes part of the same cycle of impregnation, birth, and loss. If the offspring is a male, having no purpose in an industry that exploits the female reproductive system, he is sold to become "breeding stock" – or what is called "veal." His life becomes justified by the profit derived from his death. Every year, over 800,000 male calves born to dairy cows in the U.S. are slaughtered and sold as veal – all for a product that is neither healthful nor necessary for humans to consume.

The situation is similar for dairy goats, though they have a shorter gestation period – about 5 months. They are milked for 7 to 8 months, re-bred, and milked another 2 to 3 months. Males are unwanted and sold to slaughter, and goat pregnancies are doubly problematic, as twin births are not uncommon, resulting in more unwanted lives and thus more slaughter.

Before I realized that cows had to be pregnant in order to produce milk, I also believed that consuming animals' milk didn't contribute to suffering because the cows didn't have to be killed in order for us to take her milk.

But I was wrong.

Because a cow's life is only as valuable as the offspring and amount of milk she is able to produce, when she is no longer profitable (i.e. when the costs to feed, medicate, and shelter her exceed the revenue derived from her milk output), she is sent to slaughter. Cows are impregnated beginning at about 15 months young, even though they don't reach physical maturity until they are 4 years young. By the time she is 5, after having endured three or four pregnancies (and the loss of the same number of her calves), she is sold to slaughter. Cattle have a natural life expectancy of 15 or 20 years, but dairy cows – all dairy cows – are sent to slaughter at about 4 to 5 years young[86].

Whether she is used on a small farm, an organic farm, a "humane" farm, a "family-owned" farm, an artisan farm, a whatever-it's-called-farm, she is sent to slaughter when her milk production wanes.

Whether the milk is labeled "organic," "whole," "pasteurized," "unpasteurized," "homogenized," "raw," "lactose-free," "low-fat," "2%," "1%," "skim," "fat-free," "hormone-free," or "natural," she is sent to slaughter.

More than 18% of U.S. beef comes from spent dairy cows, the majority of which is sold for fast-food hamburgers and supermarket retail[87]. In the United States, of the 9.2 million cows raised for milk, 3 million dairy cows were expected to be slaughtered in 2012[88]. Make no mistake – there is no retirement pasture for used-up cows.

As far as I'm concerned, there is simply no ethical way to keep cows or goats (or any animal) "just for their milk." You cannot stimulate lactation without pregnancy, and in order to keep milk production high and consistent, you have to keep impregnating them, while keeping their off-spring from drinking the milk that was made just for them. To fully stop the offspring from competing for what is right-fully theirs, they're sold for slaughter. To eliminate the costs of caring for "non-productive" animals, males have to be killed. Perhaps a stud or two is kept to continue impregnating the females, but you only need so many males for this purpose.

As much as we want to distance ourselves from respon-sibility and culpability, there is no such thing as a slaughter-free animal agriculture system. It is not economically viable to feed, shelter, treat, and house animals for the rest of their lives and generate no profit in return.

Dispelling the Myths

In an attempt to undermine the ethical considerations of impregnating animals for the purpose of stimulating milk production, I've heard some people *insist* that animals can be forced to lactate without having to be pregnant. *Technically*, if a human (a male or un-pregnant female) has an increase in the hormones that create milk, they, too, can lactate. But this is extremely rare. Make no mistake about it: the females used for milk production – on small farms and in large operations – impregnate their females and discard the unwanted males.

I've also heard some people insist that cows *don't* have to be impregnated again and again in order to keep her producing milk – that one pregnancy is enough to keep her lactating. Setting aside the fact that a cow is still being used, impregnated against her will, and having her offspring taken away from her, this statement reflects a misunderstanding that stems from the fact that *technically* cows (like humans) can continue giving milk for a short time after giving birth, while her offspring feeds – just like any mammal. So, again, *technically* it's true, but as time goes on, the amount of milk she produces declines. For most cows, milk production increases until about 90 days after they give birth and then slowly declines during the rest of the lactation period. That's *technically* what's going on *biologically*, but let's that's *not* what's going on in reality.

Then, there are some who assert that they know of small dairy farms who keep their calves (in the case of cows) or kids (in the case of goats). Of course, I can't speak to what a specific farm might be doing, but I would venture to guess that *if* this is the case, the farm might keep them for a short amount of time – perhaps longer than large commercial operations do – but they still eventually sell them to slaughter. There is simply no way around that. But don't take my word for it. Ask them yourself.

Even if they keep the young longer than larger operations, they still cannot let the calf drink his or her mother's milk for very long – or it defeats the entire purpose of selling her milk to humans. Some dairy farms have devised ways to prevent the calf from nursing, such as putting spiked muzzles on the calves. The muzzles have sharp barbs on the outside, so when the baby tries to nurse, he hurts his mother, and she kicks him away until he gives up. Oh, what a strange world we live in.

And we're going through all of this for what? To consume the milk of another species that even the offspring of that species stops drinking after he's weaned?

Like all mammals, at a certain age, depending on the mammal, the infant is able to move onto solid food and is weaned off of his mother's milk. In the case of humans, however, after we're weaned, we're sold the idea that we should then switch to the milk of another animal. We don't even drink our own species' milk into adulthood. At the very idea, people wrinkle up their noses in disgust. In fact, I see similar sneers at the suggestion that humans drink rat's milk or cat's milk or dog's milk. Cow's milk, goat's milk, and sheep's milk? No problem. But dog's milk? That's just disgusting!

Perhaps we have to ask ourselves why we reject consuming the lactation fluid of some species but accept consuming that of another. After all, rat, cat, and dog milk is very nutritious. Why haven't we given them a try?

Could it be because we recognize – instinctively and without marketing manipulation – that rat's milk is made for baby rats, cat's milk is made for kittens, and dog's milk is made for puppies? Could it be because we concede that animal milk is indeed very nutritious – for the offspring of the respective species?

Our bodies' physiology, in fact, supports this notion. Once we're weaned, we don't need to consume even our own species' milk, so our bodies stop producing an enzyme called lactase by the time we approach the age of weaning – at about 4 or 5 years old. Lactase is the enzyme that enables us digest lactose, which is the sugar in the milk of mammals, including humans. In other words, by the time we should be weaned, our bodies don't make this enzyme anymore. Although some people around the world adapted genetically to continue consuming animal milk without discomfort, they're the exception and not the rule. A huge percentage of the world's population suffer from what is called "lactose intolerance," experiencing gas, bloating, abdominal cramping, and diarrhea. According to the National Institutes of Health and U.S. National Library of Medicine, approximately 65% of the world's population has reduced ability to digest lactose after infancy[89].

The goat's milk industry has capitalized on this by targeting "lactose-intolerant" people in their marketing campaigns, purporting its milk to have lower amounts of lactose than cow's milk. And it's true: goat's milk has 6 percent less lactose than cow's milk. Six percent.

The bottom line is that lactose intolerance is not a disorder. It's normal!

We're not *supposed* to be consuming lactose once we're weaned. Rather than labeling the majority with a disorder, it would be more accurate to say that the minority – those whose bodies have developed to digest lactose – have "lactase persistence." If you want true lactose-free milk, drink that made from plants, which has been around for centuries and varies according to where you are in the world. Though water is really the only beverage we have a physiological need for (beyond mother's milk when we're young), it is certainly convenient and tasty to be able to make creamy, nutrient-rich milk from nuts (almonds, hazelnuts, peanuts, cashews), grains (oats and rice), legumes (soybeans and peanuts), and seeds (coconut, hemp, and sunflower). Many of these milks are now available commercially, and most can be easily made at home.

Skipping the middle cow and the middle goat is health- and life-enhancing for everyone, including the cows. We have no nutritional requirement for cow's or goat's milk, sheep's milk or buffalo milk, camel's milk or dog's milk, but we do have an ethical imperative to make choices that create as little harm as possible.

Is Honey Vegan?

A great debate rages over whether honey is vegan or not, and I confess, I don't quite understand what all the fuss is about. Honey is made by the animals, for the animals – not for me – and so, by definition it's not vegan.

Some people feel that honey is the deal breaker for people – that many who would consider being vegan would just change their minds upon realizing they'd have to "give up honey, too." Honestly, I don't think that's what keeps people from becoming vegan. If it weren't honey, it would be something else. I just don't believe that people are one small step away from being vegan but then say, "Oh –I couldn't eat honey either? Well, just forget the whole thing."

Another aspect of the honey issue is the lingering debate as to whether keeping bees constitutes cruelty, or whether bees really are harmed when their food is taken. As a result, some people argue that including honey in the fold of products that vegans avoid makes veganism seem difficult, unreasonable, rigid, or impossible. I just don't agree. If someone is already resistant to being vegan, then they will make that same argument about other animal products, too.

To me, the bottom line is that honey is not made for me; the bees make it for themselves as a source of food, and it's just not something I eat.

And besides, honey fills no nutritional need, and in fact, infants under 12 months should not even consume honey. Their digestive systems are not yet able to handle the bacteria in honey, and they may develop botulism as a result. Honey is just one of many liquid sweeteners; it's not manna from the heavens. The people who sell honey and its by-product "royal jelly" (secreted from the heads of bees to feed their new queen) will tell you it's a "wonder" food, which is ridiculous. We have no more need to consume the regurgitated food of bees than we do to consume the colostrum of cows, which is also sold in health food stores with promises of optimal health.

As for matching the texture and sweetness of honey, frankly, it's probably the easiest switcheroo you can make. Agave nectar is a wonderful plant-based liquid sweetener that has the viscosity and flavor of honey. It comes from a cactus-like plant, and if you've ever had tequila, you've had agave. For baking, you can use it for such desserts as baklava, or use it to sweeten tea. Of course, other liquid sweeteners include maple syrup, rice syrup, molasses, sorghum syrup, and barley malt, but we don't have any nutritional need for any of them either.

Although many of these are touted as health food, just keep in mind that they're all sweeteners. But when we want them as a treat, at least we have many choices in the plant kingdom and can live without the *one* in the animal kingdom. As I've said before, if someone tells me that they could stop eating everything but X (which is usually cheese, but if it's honey, I'd have the same response), I'd say great – then stop eating everything but honey – at least for now. Do everything you can, but *don't do nothing because you can't do everything. Do something. Anything!*

What Do Vegans Feed Their Cats and Dogs?

Once they become vegan, many people begin thinking about the diet of their dogs and cats. With their own diets reflecting compassion and optimum nutrition, they're naturally reluctant to support the slaughter industry by feeding their dogs and cats meat. It's a dilemma for many of us, and I have just one piece of advice: adopt a bunny. They eat lots of produce, and you don't have to worry about this issue at all (plus they make fabulous companions)!

Would that it were that simple.

I want to make it clear that there are many schools of thought about the best diet for our beloved companion animals. Ultimately, you will make the decision that best suits your individual animal. What I want to offer are my thoughts about whether dogs and cats can thrive on a plant-based diet.

In short, dogs – as natural omnivores – thrive on a plant-based diet; cats – as obligate carnivores – don't. Some dogs may have issues with allergens such as corn, soy, wheat, and gluten that are in commercial dog foods, so that's just a matter of finding the right food if that issue arises. But in general, vegan dogs do really well, and any vet who tells you otherwise is simply misinformed. There are a number of commercial vegan dog foods on the market, but of course, whenever you're making food changes in your dog's diet, you'll want to transition him or her slowly, incorporating the new food into his or her regular food little by little.

While there are many anecdotal tales of cats thriving on vegetarian and vegan diets, let's just say I'm not convinced – based on my own research and experience. Cats are physiologically built as carnivores and have very high protein requirements. They do not require plant products in their diet, though they do tend to consume some when they eat the stomach contents of their prey. Offering cats some veggie food is fine, but the foundation of their diet – at least 75 percent – should be animal-based. Making their diet 25 percent vegan is one way to compromise – enabling you to give your cats what they need to be healthy, but also cut down on the amount of meat you're buying.

One of the potential problems for vegan cats is the risk of what's called Feline Urologic Syndrome or feline urinary tract disease, which occurs when crystals form in the bladder and are unable to pass through the urethra. It's more common in males because their urethras are narrower than that of females, and it's fatal if not caught. A 100-percent vegan diet – even using the commercial cat food that's supplemented with taurine and other essential amino acids – often means that their urine is more alkaline than acidic, which can lead to the formation of crystals.

I feed my cats only canned food, and my main criteria are that it not contain byproducts or grains. A lot of the cheaper, lower-grade brands rely on byproducts (such as U.S. Department of Agriculture grade 4-D meat, which stands for dead, dying, disabled and diseased animals) as well as filler in the form of corn, which is difficult for many cats to ingest. For what it's worth, my cats eat only fish and not land animals, but to the aquatic animals, I'm aware that doesn't really mean much.

Drawing the Line

Living with integrity in a world that seems to value convenience and pleasure over ethics can be challenging at best, and since we can't be perfect, we find ourselves having to draw a line somewhere; After all, the rubber in my car tires have the remnants of animals in them; I kill insects every time I walk on the ground or drive my car; many municipal water systems use animal bones as filtering agents; and white sugar is sometimes refined through activated charcoal, most of which comes from animal bones. Clearly, we have to find a line to draw, or we'll drive ourselves crazy. It's the nature of living in an imperfect world.

But even with all of our imperfections, there is so much we can do to reduce violence and suffering. When compassion – and not perfection – is our end, the possibilities for creating a non-violent world are endless.

CHAPTER 7:

THE MYTH OF THE PERFECT VEGAN: INTENTION NOT PERFECTION

When you become vegan, you inevitably receive questions from people all around you – strangers, friends, co-workers, family members – and, unfortunately, some of them may be antagonistic. Some people may try to undermine or find fault with your choice, some may challenge the entire concept of being vegan. Because many people mistakenly believe that being vegan is about being perfect, they may accuse vegans of being hypocrites and sometimes don't hesitate to point out all the areas where vegans are imperfect.

This pressure might not even come from others; it might come from *you*. Perhaps while striving to do your best, you've accidentally eaten something that wasn't vegan and feel bad for doing so.

Once you look at the world through this vegan lens, you notice animal products in things you never even thought of before. You feel guilty, you feel overwhelmed, and you feel judged by everyone around you for "not doing it right" or for "not being perfect."

Let me assuage your fears: there is no such thing as a certified vegan, and if perfection and purity is what you're trying to attain in a world that is by its nature imperfect, then I'm afraid you'll be gravely disappointed. I cannot emphasize this enough: being vegan is not an end in itself; it's a *means* to an end, and if we forget this, then we're missing the entire point of what it means to be vegan, whether we're doing it from a health or ethical perspective – or both.

Unfortunately, I think this expectation of perfection is what stops many people from even giving veganism a try. They're afraid they're going to be expected to change everything in one fell swoop, and their fear is justified when they proudly declare to someone that they're vegan, and they're met with a smug reminder that the shoes they're wearing are made of leather. "Ha!" they seem to say, deriving pleasure in catching you at not being perfect after all.

Whenever I've been in the situation where it seems someone's trying to *catch* me, I'm aware of what a great privilege and responsibility it is to help change the perception of what it means to be vegan. Unabashedly, I admit that I'm far from perfect, that I'm doing the best I can, and that I'm trying to make a difference where I'm able. Being vegan is not about being perfect; it's about reducing suffering when and where I can.

When people dismiss veganism as attainable or unrealistic, remind them that not doing *anything* because we can't do *everything* makes absolutely no sense. *Don't do nothing because you can't do everything. Do something. Anything.*

What about the leather couch and shoes or wool coat you bought in your pre-vegan ("pregan") days? Some new vegans simply can't stand the thought of wearing any of the animal products that once gave them so much pleasure, and so they slowly replace them with the array of beautiful skin-free products available. Most people can't afford to do this all at once, and so they do it over time. That's *fine*. You do what you can as you're able.

Being vegan is about creating compassion and not creating harm whenever it's practical and possible to do so. So when you're faced with this dilemma, the question to ask is: "How does keeping this leather couch (for instance) contribute to animal cruelty today?" Or flip it around: "How does getting rid of it *help* animals today?" As it becomes difficult to even have the couch in your home, then sell it and save for a new one. Or sell it, and donate the money to an animal organization. Give it away or have it re-upholstered.

You can even keep it. It's up to you.

The most counterproductive response is to beat yourself up for once having purchased these things. We make what we think are the best decisions with the information we have at the time; as we grow and learn, we can strive to make the most compassionate decisions possible.

Just keep in mind that being vegan is about intention – not perfection.

Accidents Happen

Although vegans do their best to avoid animal products, it can be difficult (and is unrealistic) to try and shun every animal-derived ingredient, some of which may be hidden. Keeping in mind your goals – whether you're trying to avoid contributing to violence towards animals, or to eat only life-enhancing rather than life-taking foods, or to reduce the use of the Earth's resources, or all of these things – will help keep things in perspective when you accidentally eat something that has gelatin or eggs.

Here's how I handle that situation: I write it off as an accident, and I move on. Every vegan I know has bitten into a sandwich that contained some non-vegan ingredient. Even in vegan-friendly restaurants, I've witnessed vegan friends chew on what they thought was tofu but turned out to be a chicken's breast. Twice, I've even eaten what I realized was pork after I swallowed – once in a Mexican restaurant and once in an Asian restaurant.

Although it's not pleasant, and it can be emotionally upsetting, accidents happen. I certainly recommend talking to the server and telling them about the mistake, and competent management will apologize and try to rectify the situation; but in terms of dwelling on it, there's no point. Take whatever lessons can be gleaned from the experience and apply them to future scenarios.

The Vegan in the Room

I was once asked by someone if I'm a "hardcore" vegan. I asked her what she meant. She said "Do you ever cheat? Do you ever sneak a piece of cheese or are you hardcore?" I told her that if by "hardcore" she meant "Am I consistent?" then yes, I suppose I'm hardcore.

For me, being vegan is about expansiveness and openness. Not restriction. Not limitation. Not rules. Not doctrine. It's one of the reasons I correct people when they say "Oh you can't have that because you're vegan." Of course I *can* have it. I'm not *forbidden* to eat animals or their secretions. The point is that I don't *want* to eat animals and their secretions. And there is freedom and serenity in that choice.

For me, being vegan is about living my life with integrity and compassion, knowing that every decision I make is done so with the intention of not contributing to the suffering and exploitation of human and non-human animals.

I think people aren't used to other people walking the talk. We all say we have certain values, but that doesn't mean we necessarily reflect them in our behavior. Being vegan is about reflecting our compassion and desire for health in our actions. It doesn't mean we're going to succeed all the time, but just having the intention means we will manifest these values more often than not.

We live in a world that seeks to encourage empathy, kindness, and compassion in children but seems suspicious of these same values in adults. We live in a world where human privilege and the desire for convenience and pleasure drive the socially sanctioned use and abuse of billions and billions of nonhuman animals. We live in a world where it's considered normal to champion this and radical to oppose it.

The excuses people come up with to justify tradition and habit can range from the absurd to the offensive, and new vegans are often caught off guard by the defensiveness that seems to be directed toward what to them is simply a healthful, kind way for them to live. Even when the reaction isn't hostile, vegans are often asked to defend how and why they eat the way they do. Although non-vegans are never asked to explain why they eat meat, dairy, and eggs, the most common question meat-eaters ask those who don't eat animals is "Why are you vegan?"

This can be difficult for some people to reconcile; not everyone wants to have to answer to their food choices every time they sit down to eat. And I understand that. Not everyone who is vegan is necessarily an activist. But the truth is whether we like it or not, if we're the vegan someone meets, if we're the vegan someone comes to, we represent *all vegans*; we become *the vegan ambassador* - the "vegan in the room." I realize that puts a lot of pressure on vegans, but with so many myths perpetuated about and against vegan-ism, if we brush off people's questions or answer without patience and understanding, then we may be squandering an opportunity to show how positive and healthful this way of living really is.

We certainly don't have to become experts in nutrition, anthropology, animal husbandry, or the culinary arts, but I do believe we have an obligation to speak our truth when someone asks us why we're vegan – not only for ourselves (and for the animals, if that's part of your story) but also for the benefit of the person asking.

For instance, when someone asks me why I'm vegan, personally, I don't spout off all the statistics and studies that support the benefits of a vegan diet – and there are plenty. When someone asks me why I'm vegan, I tell *my* story, *my* truth, *my authentic* reason for being vegan, which is simply that I don't want to contribute to suffering and violence. Period. Especially where I have the power to do so. Nobody can take away *my* truth, *my* story! I don't have to worry about someone arguing with me and saying "that's not true" or "you're wrong." No one can say that when I speak my truth. From there, the rest is not mine. In speaking my truth, I may inspire others to act on their own values, but if they don't, that's not mine to worry about.

Let me put it another way – though this may surprise you – my *intention* in the work I do is not to "make people vegan." My intention is not to change someone's mind. My intention is not to *make* people do something. My intention is not to win an argument. My intention is to raise awareness about the violence inherent in a mindset and culture that brings animals into this world only to kill them. My intention is to be a voice for the voiceless – for the animals who need advocates to speak for them. My intention is to give people the tools they need to live according to their own values of compassion and wellness.

My intention is to inspire – not convert. There is a huge difference.

I believe we're here to be teachers for one another, and I'm grateful for my role as a conduit, but that's all any of us are. I believe *intention* is everything, and when our intention is simply to plant seeds and remain unattached to the outcome, we can't **but** succeed in having a pleasant and effective dialogue with people who inquire about our lifestyle (and they *will* inquire).

Whenever we're answering questions about being vegan, it helps to have a clear intention, and I think if our intention is "to speak the truth" rather than "to convert someone," we will be very effective spokespeople for this incredible way of living.

I think being focused on intention rather than outcome also takes a lot of the pressure off. In other words, don't feel that you have to have all the answers or that you have to speak so eloquently on behalf of a vegan lifestyle that you wind up not speaking at all. In *your* truth lies your eloquence. In *your* story lies someone else's. But in order to tell your story, you first have to remember it. And I think remembering our stories is key to staying humble, feeling confidence, and inspiring others.

Remembering Our Stories

Many a vegan has been in a situation where all they have to say is "I'm vegan" for feathers to fly. I believe we're all mirrors to one another, and at any given moment, we reflect back to one another something we may need to look at in ourselves. Sometimes, non-vegans feel threatened in the presence of a vegan because the mirror held up to them may reflect something they're uncomfortable with in their own behavior. Maybe they want to stop eating animals but haven't brought themselves to do it. Maybe they feel guilty. Whatever it is, I call this dynamic the result of being "the vegan in the room." Without even intending to, the vegan can change the mood of a room without ever saying a word.

But just as non-vegans need to confront this reflection and choose to either accept or reject what comes up for them, so, too, do vegans need to look in the mirror when we meet someone who is still eating animal meat, milk, and eggs and look squarely at what comes up for us. Is it impatience? Judgment? Self-righteousness? Arrogance? All of the above?

These reactions are understandable. When you stop eating animals, you become keenly aware of how often people are eating this stuff, and it can be very upsetting. You're look at the world through a new lens, and you want everyone to see what you see. But if we try to force them to, I don't think we'll be very effective. If we're pushy, hostile, angry, passive-aggressive, self-righteous, or arrogant, we *will* turn people away. *That* I can guarantee.

We absolutely have to remember that we were once unaware, that we once ate animals, that we once may have made excuses for eating them and perhaps even made fun of "those crazy vegans." In forgetting our own stories and our own process, we lose our humility and the ability to be effective, compassionate spokespeople for this wonderful way of life.

Remember your story, and tell your story. Connect with other vegans – either online or in person, and ask them to tell *their* stories. Creating a community of like-minded people is vital to remaining a joyful vegan, but finding common ground with people who aren't where you're at is also essential.

Looking Forward – Not Backward

When animals were first herded and domesticated for human use and consumption about 10,000 years ago[90], they became the alternatives to the plant foods that were then the foundation of the human diet. While humans ate mostly small animals and little of them, plant foods played the larger role. Thousands of years later, entrenched in an archaic animal-based agricultural system controlled by those who benefit financially, the roles have reversed. Animal-based products are dominant in most people's diets, while plant foods are regarded as side dishes or garnishes.

With a determination that belies an irrational attachment to animal flesh and fluids, I've seen otherwise sensible and sensitive people spend time and energy extolling the human history of eating and domesticating animals. Using lyrical and exalted language, they wax poetic about the virtues of animal husbandry and glorify the prehistoric hunter-gatherer, who, according to mounting anthropological evidence, was more likely a gatherer-hunter. Still, the argument goes something like this: since early humans ate animals, we're justified in continuing to eat them now.

Some contemporary food writers even charge vegetarians and vegans with turning their backs on their "evolutionary heritage," strangely perceiving Darwinian evolution as a moral system by which we should justify our actions. By eschewing meat, they say, we're "sacrificing a part of our identity." It seems to me that we have the ability and responsibility to make moral and rational decisions – not abdicate our ethics to an amoral process. Surely, our identities are defined by more than our paleontological past. And yet, determined to dwell perpetually on this past, these same people even romanticize the life of "cavemen" in order to rationalize our contemporary consumption of animals. Certainly there are lessons to learn from our human predecessors, but do we really want to use Neanderthals or Paleolithic humans as the model for our ethics? Can't we do better than that?

We often say that we want to do better than we did a generation ago, two generations ago. I presume we want to do better than we did hundreds of thousands of years ago. That's the point of being human, isn't it? To learn from our past and make better, more healthful, more compassionate choices once we know better, especially once we have the ability and opportunity to do so?

Being vegan is about choosing compassion over violence; it's not about being perfect, and it's not about being pure. It's not even about doing better than someone else. It's about doing better than we did before. And considering our history, we can only go up from here.

My hope is that we each embrace our unconditional compassion and express it unapologetically and at full throttle. Though I don't believe people wake up in the morning committed to creating as much violence and suffering as possible, I also don't believe people wake up in the morning committed to creating as much compassion, peace, and nonviolence as possible. If that were on our to-do list every day, imagine what we could accomplish. Imagine what our world would be like.

RECOMMENDED RESOURCES

Here are a number of related resources for your edification and enjoyment.

AUTHOR'S WEBSITES
www.compassionatecook.com (main website)
www.30dayveganchallenge.com (30-Day Vegan Challenge)
www.vegetarianfoodforthought.com (podcast)

HEALTH & WELLNESS
These experts specialize in the fields of research and treatment of preventable diseases. Many of them have several or seminal books, which you can find on their websites.

Caldwell Esselstyn, Jr., MD www.heartattackproof.com
T. Colin Campbell, PhD www.tcolincampbell.org
John Robbins www.johnrobbins.info
Jack Norris, RD www.veganhealth.org
Vesanto Melina, MS, RD www.nutrispeak.com
John McDougall, MD www.drmcdougall.com

Michael Greger, MD www.drgreger.org

Michael Klaper, MD www.doctorklaper.com

Joel Fuhrman, MD www.drfuhrman.com

Pam Popper, PhD, ND www.wellnessforum.com

Physicians Committee for Responsible Medicine www.pcrm.org

World Peace Diet www.worldpeacediet.com

Brenda Davis, RD www.brendadavisrd.com

Becoming Vegan by Brenda Davis and Vesanto Melina is *the* bible of vegan nutrition, and their book *Becoming Raw* answers all the questions about raw diets.

Visit www.b12.com for the most accurate testing of your vitamin B12 levels.

The Vitamin D Council has partnered with ZRT Labs to make a discounted take-home Vitamin D Test Kit that you can order at https://vitamindcouncil.zrtlab.com.

RECOMMENDED READING

Diet for a New America: How Your Food Choices Affect Your Health, Happiness and the Future of Life on Earth by John Robbins

Why We Love Dogs, Eat Pigs, and Wear Cows: An Introduction to Carnism by Melanie Joy, PhD

An Unnatural Order: Roots of Our Destruction of Nature by Jim Mason

Animal Liberation by Peter Singer

Slaughterhouse: The Shocking Story of Greed, Neglect, and Inhumane Treatment Inside the U.S. Meat Industry by Gail A. Eisnitz

Mad Cowboy: Plain Truth from the Cattle Rancher Who Won't Eat Meat by Howard Lyman

Dominion: The Power of Man, the Suffering of Animals, and the Call to Mercy by Matthew Scully

For the Prevention of Cruelty: The History and Legacy of Animal Rights Activism in the United States by Diane L. Beers

Food Politics: How the Food Industry Influences Nutrition and Health by Marion Nestle

RECOMMENDED VIEWING

The people who work undercover to get footage of the plights of animals are unsung heroes, and the best way we can honor their work is to view what they have documented via video, audio, and still photos. The following organizations have videos of undercover investigations as well as life-changing films and photographs available to view on their websites:

*The documentary "Earthlings" www.earthlings.com

*The documentaries "Peaceable Kingdom" and "The Witness" www.tribeofheart.org

*Photographer Jo-Anne McArthur www.weanimals.org

*The Humane Society of the United States www.hsus.org

*Mercy for Animals www.mercyforanimals.org

*Compassion Over Killing www.cok.net

*People for the Ethical Treatment of Animals www. peta.org

*Our Hen House www.ourhenhouse.org

VEGAN DOG FOOD AND TREATS

V-Dog www.v-dog.com
Evolution Diet www.petfoodshop.com
Natural Life Pet Products www.nlpp.com
Natural Balance www.naturalbalanceinc.com
Nature's Recipe www.naturesrecipe.com
PetGuard www.petguard.com
Boston Baked Bonz www.bostonbakedbonz.com
Vegan Cats (for supplements, info, and dog food) www.vegancats.com

SUPPLEMENTS

Dr. Fuhrman's multivitamins, vitamin D, omega 3's (called DHA Purity), and other supplements for various stages of life are sold at www.compassionatecooks.com/supplements

ACKNOWLEDGEMENTS

The making of a book starts with a seed that grows with the help of many hands, and I'm incredibly thankful for everyone who helped my idea for this book germinate, take root, and blossom.

First and foremost, I'm immensely grateful to my husband David Goudreau, my beautiful partner in life, love, laughter, compassion, and dance! Every day with you is better than the one before.

I'm blessed to be surrounded by so many loving friends (you know who you are) and supportive family members, and I'm kept sane and productive by a number of people whose skills and shared commitment to compassion help me accomplish my mission, particularly Tim Anderson, Alexander Gray, David Cabrera, Robin Brande, Jim Kenney, Amanda Mitchell, Mackenzie Mount, Florian Radke, Brighde Reed, Brett Renville, Aaron Weinstein, and Blake Wiers. I value their perspective, intuition, and expertise so very much, and I've quite come to rely on their advice and support.

I am so incredibly thankful to have the honor and privilege of hearing from so many remarkable people whose eyes and hearts have been opened and who let me be part of their journey. Thank you to everyone who has ever listened to my podcast, read my books, used my recipes, watched my videos, or attended my talks. You are the reason I awaken with hope every day.

Thank you to each and every person who uses his or her voice to speak for those who have no voice. Whether you do it formally as part of a larger organization or on your own as a grassroots activist, every seed you plant contributes to the compassionate world we all envision.

And what a blessing it is to live in the company of cats. Charlie and Michiko bring me immense joy every moment of every day, and courageous Simon, magical Schuster, and sweet Cassandra continue to live in my heart.

My greatest inspirations are the non-human animals of the world. I dedicate my work to them, and I look forward to the day when online dictionaries don't try to replace my use of "he," "she," and "who" with "it" and "that" when referring to these beautiful, sensitive, living, feeling beings.

ABOUT THE AUTHOR

Colleen Patrick-Goudreau has dedicated her life to empowering people to make informed food choices, to debunking myths about veganism, to being a voice for animals, and to giving people the tools and resources they need to live according to their own values of compassion and wellness. Using her unique blend of passion, humor, and common sense, Colleen adeptly addresses the ethical, social, and practical aspects of a compassionate lifestyle.

A powerful writer, talented chef, and exhilarating speaker, she is the author of six books, including the award-winning *The Joy of Vegan Baking*, *The Vegan Table*, *Color Me Vegan*, and *Vegan's Daily Companion*. With a command of traditional and new media, Colleen is the creator of the popular online multimedia program, The 30-Day Vegan Challenge; the host and producer of the life-changing podcast Vegetarian Food for Thought; and she delivers inspiring lectures around the country. She has appeared on the Food Network and PBS and is a contributor to National Public Radio and *The Christian Science Monitor*.

BIBLIOGRAPHY

Chapter 2: Defining Vegan

[1] http://www.foodsforlife.org.uk/people/Donald-Watson-Vegan/Donald-Watson.html

[2] http://www.foodsforlife.org.uk/people/Donald-Watson-Vegan/Donald-Watson.html

Chapter 3: Why Vegan? Pick a Reason – Any Reason

[3] http://www.cdc.gov/foodsafety/facts.html#what

[4] http://www.cdc.gov/foodborneburden/2011-foodborne-estimates.html

[5] http://www.aphis.usda.gov/wildlife_damage/prog_data/2011_prog_data/PDR_G/Basic_Tables_PDR_G/Table%20G_ShortReport.pdf

[6] http://www.greenpeace.org/usa/en/campaigns/victories/oceans-victories/

[7] http://www.greenpeace.org/international/en/campaigns/oceans/bycatch/?accept=18fe3ea3e2b342aa4bfeed2cccaf63a6

8   http://www.pewenvironment.org/news-room/
    reports/the-future-of-sharks-a-review-of-action-and-
    inaction-8589941475

9   http://today.duke.edu/2004/03/seaturtle_0304.html

10 http://www.dfo-mpo.gc.ca/misc/seal_briefing_e.htm

11 http://www.nefsc.noaa.gov/publications/tm/tm205/
    pdfs/214HarpS.pdf

12 http://www.fao.org/docrep/010/a0701e/a0701e00.htm

13 http://www.fao.org/newsroom/en/news/
    2006/1000448/index.html

14 http://pubs.acs.org/doi/full/10.1021/es702969f

15 http://www.eatright.org/Media/content.aspx?
    id=1233#.URQxV6V8ujF

16 ftp://ftp.fao.org/docrep/fao/010/a0701e/a0701e02.pdf

17 http://www.ncbi.nlm.nih.gov/pmc/articles/
    PMC2367646/

18 http://www.humanesociety.org/animals/cows/

19 http://www.fsis.usda.gov/Fact_Sheets/Beef_from_
    Farm_to_Table/index.asp

20 Marji Beach, Advocacy & Education Director at Animal
    Place, http://animalplace.org/

21 http://www.ers.usda.gov/data-products/livestock-
    meat-domestic-data.aspx#26084

22 http://www.fsis.usda.gov/Fact_Sheets/Veal_from_
    Farm_to_Table/index.asp

23 http://www.ers.usda.gov/data-products/livestock-
    meat-domestic-data.aspx#26084

24 Marji Beach, Advocacy & Education Director at Animal
    Place, http://animalplace.org/

25 http://www.fsis.usda.gov/Fact_Sheets/Pork_From_
Farm_to_Table/index.asp

26 Marji Beach, Advocacy & Education Director at Animal
Place, http://animalplace.org/

27 http://www.ers.usda.gov/data-products/livestock-
meat-domestic-data.aspx#26084

28 http://www.fsis.usda.gov/Fact_Sheets/Chicken_
from_Farm_To_Table/index.asp

29 http://www.fsis.usda.gov/Fact_Sheets/Chicken_
from_Farm_To_Table/index.asp

30 Marji Beach, Advocacy & Education Director at Animal
Place, http://animalplace.org/

31 http://www.ers.usda.gov/data-products/livestock-
meat-domestic-data.aspx#26084

32 http://www.gpo.gov/fdsys/pkg/CFR-2012-title9-
vol2/xml/CFR-2012-title9-vol2-part313.xml

33 http://www.fsis.usda.gov/Fact_Sheets/Turkey_from_
Farm_to_Table/index.asp

34 Marji Beach, Advocacy & Education Director at Animal
Place, http://animalplace.org/

35 http://www.ers.usda.gov/data-products/livestock-
meat-domestic-data.aspx#26084

36 http://www.fsis.usda.gov/Fact_Sheets/Duck_&_
Goose_from_Farm_to_Table/index.asp

37 Marji Beach, Advocacy & Education Director at Animal
Place, http://animalplace.org/

38 http://www.humanesociety.org/news/resources/
research/stats_slaughter_totals.html

39 http://www.fsis.usda.gov/FACTSheets/Duck_&_Goose_from_Farm_to_Table/index.asp

40 Marji Beach, Advocacy & Education Director at Animal Place, http://animalplace.org/

41 http://www.ers.usda.gov/data-products/livestock-meat-domestic-data.aspx#26147

42 http://www.fsis.usda.gov/Fact_Sheets/Goat_from_Farm_to_Table/index.asp

43 Marji Beach, Advocacy & Education Director at Animal Place, http://animalplace.org/

44 http://usda.mannlib.cornell.edu/MannUsda/viewDocumentInfo.do?documentID=1096

45 http://www.fsis.usda.gov/Fact_Sheets/Rabbit_from_Farm_to_Table/index.asp

46 Marji Beach, Advocacy & Education Director at Animal Place, http://animalplace.org/

47 http://www.aphis.usda.gov/animal_health/emergingissues/industryprofiles/industryprofiles.shtml

48 http://www.fsis.usda.gov/Fact_Sheets/Lamb_from_Farm_to_Table/index.asp

49 Marji Beach, Advocacy & Education Director at Animal Place, http://animalplace.org/

50 http://www.ers.usda.gov/data-products/livestock-meat-domestic-data.aspx#26084

51 Marji Beach, Advocacy & Education Director at Animal Place, http://animalplace.org/

52 http://www.ers.usda.gov/data-products/livestock-meat-domestic-data.aspx#26147

53 www.aphis.usda.gov/animal_health/nahms/downloads/Demographics2011.pdf

54 http://www.gao.gov/products/GAO-11-228
55 Marji Beach, Advocacy & Education Director at Animal Place, http://animalplace.org/
56 http://www.humanesociety.org/issues/horse_slaughter/facts/transport_to_slaughter_092909.html
57 "Livestock Confinement Dusts and Gases." Iowa State University Extension. 1992. http://nasdonline.org/static_content/documents/1627/d001501.pdf (5/27/10
58 http://foodispower.org/factory_farm_workers.php
59 http://www.ufw.org/_page.php?menu=research&inc=history/09.html
60 http://www.fsis.usda.gov/FACTSheets/Parasites_and_Foodborne_Illness/index.asp
61 http://www.ncbi.nlm.nih.gov/pubmed/19562864
62 http://www.bcbst.com/MPManual/HW.htm
63 http://nhlbisupport.com/bmi/
64 http://www.nhlbi.nih.gov/guidelines/obesity/e_txtbk/txgd/4142.htm
65 http://www.acefitness.org/acefit/healthy_living_tools_content.aspx?id=2
66 http://www.nhlbi.nih.gov/hbp/detect/categ.htm
67 http://www.diabetes.org/diabetes-basics/diabetes-statistics/
68 http://www.mayoclinic.com/health/prediabetes/DS00624/DSECTION=tests-and-diagnosis
69 http://www.cdc.gov/cholesterol/facts.htm
70 http://www.judgerc.org/nutrition/health_questionnaire/health_goals.html

71 http://www.mayoclinic.com/health/triglycerides/
    CL00015
72 http://www.medicinenet.com/homocysteine/article.
    htm
73 http://www.veganhealth.org/articles/bones
74 http://www.veganhealth.org/articles/vitaminb12

Chapter 6: Drawing the Line – How Vegan Is Vegan?

75 http://www.epa.gov/agriculture/ag101/printpoultry.
    html
76 www.ca.uky.edu/smallflocks/Factsheets/**Sexing_
    day_old_chicks**.pdf
77 www.humanesociety.org/assets/pdfs/farm/welfare_
    egg.pdf
78 http://www.fsis.usda.gov/Fact_Sheets/Focus_On_
    Shell_Eggs/index.asp#2
79 Marji Beach, Advocacy & Education Director at Animal
    Place, http://animalplace.org/
80 Marji Beach, Advocacy & Education Director at Animal
    Place, http://animalplace.org/
81 www.humanesociety.org/assets/pdfs/farm/welfare_
    egg.pdf
82 Marji Beach, Advocacy & Education Director at Animal
    Place, http://animalplace.org/
83 Marji Beach, Advocacy & Education Director at Animal
    Place, http://animalplace.org/
84 Marji Beach, Advocacy & Education Director at Animal
    Place, http://animalplace.org/

85   http://classes.ansci.illinois.edu/ansc438/lactation/dryperiod.html

86   http://www.epa.gov/oecaagct/ag101/dairyphases.html

87   http://www.cggc.duke.edu/environment/valuechainanalysis/CGGC_BeefDairyReport_2-16-09.pdf

88   http://dairybusiness.com/seo/headline.php?title=2012-u-s-dairy-cow-slaughter-on-pace-to-hit-3&date=2012-12-17&table=headlines

89   http://ghr.nlm.nih.gov/condition/lactose-intolerance

Chapter 7: The Myth of the Perfect Vegan: Intention Not Perfection

90   http://courses.biology.utah.edu/carrier/3320/readings/westerndiet.pdf